Ana

Thank you for your kindness & positive vibes when I

Awaken to Natural Health

visit Barnes & Noble

Katina Love

Yours in Wellness!

KLove

Awaken To Natural Health

Published and distributed both in the United States and internationally by the author. For information including usage rights, publication and direct correspondence with the author:

Visit YouTube Channel: **Awakening with Katina Love Wellness**

Love@KatinaLove.com
www.KatinaLove.com

This print edition was compiled, edited and formatted by Dean's List Publishers, a division of Dean's List Communications.

For direct correspondence with them:

Dean's List Publishers
2632 S. Rochester Rd, #71181
Rochester Hills, MI 48307
deanslistpublishers@gmail.com

Lotus Life

Cover Photo Credit: Paul Heussenstamm

DISCLAIMER: This material is for informational and educational purposes only. The author does not claim suggestions, products mentioned or services recommended herein will prevent, treat or cure any specific conditions or disease. The author and publisher accept no responsibilities for any consequences however adverse or great; as a result of reading what's shared herein. The opinions and beliefs shared here are those of the author including experiences, research and studies. Always consult with your inner guidance (You) and your doctor before making changes concerning your health.

Contents

Acknowledgments

The following lists of individuals have served as inspirations and motivators for both my work as a Natural Wellness Coach and to write this book!

James Harvey, your encouragement & living example of what good health looks like. Thank you for teaching me raw food dishes & how to be creative with them.

Louise L. Hay, from your book, "You Can Heal Your Life", & your intuitive nature, I have drawn great encouragement to make affirmations and wellness part of my everyday life.

Stacey A. Kimbrell, your tenacity has shown me the need for the work we do in the world!

Dr. George King, your teachings about the importance of deep breathing allowed me to experience and add this important component to my lifestyle.

Ellen Livingston, the day I finally woke up and said, "Ok, I will do this." was when I was sitting in your raw food class ! Thanks for sharing your journey!

Joy Malone, Thanks for introducing me to Young Living Essentials Oils! This & your friendships are true invaluable gifts to me!

Gerson Martinez, yours is a shining example of being pure, authentic & your willingness to share your natural health and positive thinking lifestyle with me was a true gift.

Kevin Trudeau, your book, "Natural Cures They Don't Want You to Know About", introduced me to natural remedies which are readily and easily accessible.

And to others too numerous to mention -- thank you and blessings upon you! -- KL

My Passion For Wellness

I have been on a health and wellness journey and helping others for more than 11 years, and have helped to change the lives of many people. My mission is to help you ***Awaken to the Natural and Healthy things Mother Earth has to offer!*** I have done research on and experienced the benefits of essential oils, super foods, liquid herbal extracts, sea vegetables, algae, sea weeds, vitamins, minerals, fruit, vegetables, roots, nuts, seeds. I personally have experienced how they can benefit the human body. I have been successful with releasing ailments such as asthma, allergies, and anemia from my body; just to name a few.

I have also been successful with improving my immune system and sleep pattern, maintaining a healthy digestive system and a healthy weight. I can attribute much of my wellness success to positive thinking, prayers & affirmations, deep breathing, exercise, and sunlight and among other things, eating a diet of at least 50% raw, organic foods.

Promoting the use of natural-toxic free skin and body care, hair care, and household products; is also another one of my passions. I am affiliated with companies that produce natural products that are non-toxic and better for health only after testing and trying the products for myself. These companies continually demonstrate to me a care about humanity and the wellbeing of all.

I travel nationwide, to share my message of wellness. I give workshops and seminars, to help others improve their health, by adopting and maintaining a lifestyle that is as natural as possible!

In this book, I share my experiences and knowledge in efforts to help others prevent unnecessary suffering from toxic elements in modern society.

This book contains information that suggests a lifestyle change! It will be helpful for anyone, whether you want to practice prevention or if there is ANY dis-ease or discomfort in the body. Your body is intelligent and was designed to heal and repair itself, provided you are giving the proper things it needs. The saying that goes "You are what you eat." is literally true! Give your body the healthy things it needs and you will reap the rewards!

No matter what your situation is, there is still hope! When we change our mind-set and diet, we change our lives! Your Whole body will become Balanced when the necessary changes are made. In other words, you can release any type of ailment or dis-ease as a result and or maintain a healthy body.

My experience with Optimal Health is Whole-body wellness and includes emotional, spiritual, mental and physical well-being. I have also learned, the easier and more loving we are towards ourselves, the easier it is to make necessary changes.

I'd like you to look at your relationship when it comes to food. Perhaps we should look at the core reason why we consume food. Food is fuel we use to provide the cells in our bodies nourishment; so that our bodies can function properly ...however, at the same time our food should be enjoyed!

Our cells are what determine if we will have good eyesight, a healthy liver, heart, bones, teeth, brain and so forth. If we feed our bodies junk, we will produce weak cells and organs may not perform at Optimal level. If, however, we feed our cells healthy, wholesome natural foods, we have a better chance of building and maintaining healthy, strong organs that work properly and having Optimal health! Also I have found the most benefit is to only eat when I am hungry.

Katina Love
June 2015

How I Awakened to Natural Wellness

Along my journey to wellness, I had some valuable lessons along the way! As an adult, I have learned through trial and error, what is best for the body to achieve and maintain Optimal Health! Based on my own experience, my focus in this section is to help you see alternatives, according to what I experienced as a child, adolescent and adult. What I have learned from these experiences is …life is a precious gift and we should live each waking moment in GRATITUDE. These experiences built my passion and compelling mission to educate others on how to TAKE CONTROL of their own health! You are the only person who can take better care of your health. It starts with you!

Ancient History about Medicine from Nature

I personally believe, everything we need for our bodies to Function Properly, Feel Energized, Be Well, Have Vitality & Longevity, is in nature; *along with prayer, meditation, love, fresh air and so forth.* It's a knowing that I have deep within me. What we need for our health can be found in nature! The messages have been given throughout the ancient scriptures! **Gen. 1:29** *"I give you every seed-bearing plant on the face of the whole earth & every tree that has fruit with seed in it. They will be yours for food."*

Another one is: **Ezekiel 47:12,** *"By the river on its bank, on one side and on the other, will grow all kinds of trees for food. Their leaves will not wither and their fruit will not fail. They will bear every month because* *their water flows from the sanctuary, and their fruit will be for food and their leaves for healing."* There are so many more!

I truly believe my past experience with these illnesses was caused by a combination of malnourishment, emotional stress, processed foods and toxic chemicals. When these were eliminated, my life changed and now I am on a healthy path of wellness and vitality!

Forgiveness Contributed To My Healing

My upbringing was dysfunctional, due to an alcoholic father in the home. This did affect me emotionally, mentally and physically. One thing that did work in my favor was, after all the things I experienced with my dad, directly or indirectly; I always loved him unconditionally, totally forgave him and I have always been close to him in relationship.

I share this to let you know of the power of forgiveness, how it can allow you freedom and good health. Forgiveness can release many illnesses that people live with. If there is anyone you need to forgive, it will improve your emotional, mental and physical health to release it, as soon as possible!

Forgiveness Exercise:

Meditate for 5 minutes and think of all the things you are Grateful for. Examples include: Your health, children, career, place to live, etc.

Now imagine yourself releasing the thing(s) you feel someone else did to you, no matter what it is.

If necessary, give them a call. If they are deceased, say ______, I forgive you, then release and forget it! There is no time like the present time.

How did this make you feel?

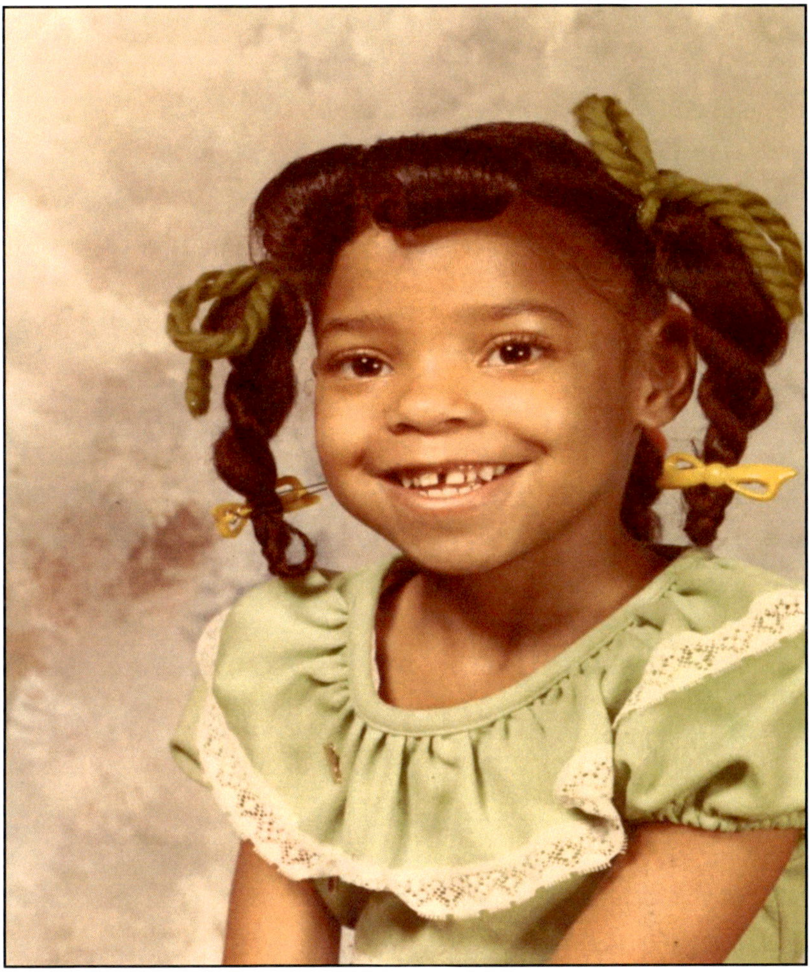

Me at Age 5

Releasing Asthma and Allergies

Children should ***never*** *breathe or come in contact with things that are unnatural!* I realized this when I became an adult and was able to release asthma and allergies on my own! If you have children, do them and yourself a favor and cease the use of cleaning products with toxic chemicals! This includes laundry detergents, dish soaps, hand soaps, lotions, deodorants, perfumes, body sprays and household cleaners. Your skin is your largest organ and whatever it comes in contact with, can enter the body through the skin and blood stream. If it would make you ill to ingest it, don't use it on your body or inside your home! Consider using all natural products instead! Also if you live in a fairly neutral environment where the air is acceptably clean; open windows as often as possible to allow fresh air in. This can possibly help everyone to breathe better and improve their well-being. The way I maintain in this area, is by using Young Living essential oils daily! Diffusing them also has many benefits. Trust me, I speak from experience!

We Need All of Our Organs

Our bodies were designed and wonderfully made in the Image of God. Our bodies are also the vehicles that house our soul and where the Divine or Spirit of God resides; as Spiritual Beings having a human experience. Therefore, the Creator knew ahead of time what it would take to have the best experience possible, while on Planet Earth. So your organs are needed in the Whole scheme of things. It does not matter if you are told, you can live without them, and you still need them to have a balanced body! When I was 17, my spleen and gall bladder were removed, so I realize how greatly they are needed.

The key is to have WHOLENESS which means to have a Healthy, Balanced Body. When the body is Balanced, Optimal Health is the result. So in order for this to be obtained, All Organs should work on Optimal Level! Keep your organs working properly now, and you can be healthy all the days of your life and keep All your organs! If it is not life threatening, you may want to take some time and do your research first for alternatives, and keep your organs!

Whenever someone is told, a particular organ should or has to be removed, consider the following: **(1)** Why? **(2)** If associated with a condition, what caused the condition? **(3)** How can the condition be corrected? **(4)** What are the alternatives (this is where research is necessary on your part, about natural alternatives)?

When organs are removed, other organs will need to compensate and do the job of its counterparts. For this reason, you want to help the other organs as much as possible!

If I could go do things differently without having surgeries, I would have! Since my spleen and gall bladder are not present. I now take supplements to make up the difference and to help the other organs work at Optimal Level.

The **spleen** is a solid organ and part of the lymphatic system and immune system. The primary functions of the spleen, is to filter blood and as part of the immune system; produce natural antibodies to keep the body strong and healthy.

When this organ is not present, my experience has been to establish a diet as clean and healthy as possible, and I also take immune building supplements. One that is very helpful is ASTRAGALUS liquid extract and I particularly like the brand **Nature's Answer.** Other things I do is drink par 'de Arco and thyme tea regularly and eat raw garlic almost daily. I also take Immune Defense capsules from time to time. All of these are Natural immune builders! Peppermint tea is also helpful.

The **gall bladder** is a hollow organ and its function is to store bile, which is a digestive juice the liver produces and it helps to break down foods that contain fat.

When this organ is not present, my experience has been to eat Organic Dark leafy greens and every so often I take the supplement **Dandelion Root** herbal extract, which is very helpful. I have found, that dandelion root helps the liver to breakdown fats along with the bile it produces and the indications are: my stool is the right color (mid-brown). If I eat mostly raw plant based foods, it might be more (dark green). One more thing I do when consuming a full course meal is to take **digestive enzymes.** When I take both dandelion root extract and digestive enzymes, I rotate between the two of them.

So, if you also had your gall bladder removed, think twice before you eat a hand full of nuts or other foods containing fats. You may need assistance with breaking it down to be more easily digestible! Eating an apple on an empty stomach before your meal is another helpful option. Have your digestive enzymes with you at all times!

How I Corrected Anemia

This can be easily corrected. The main mineral I increased was Iron along with other vital minerals! When your diet is balanced, your body will become balanced! Also, by eating Raw, Organic dark leafy greens & salads, beets (which is a root), raw and organic fruit, variety of veggies, and Whole Food multi-vitamin. That was it! Remember the goal is to make wellness a way of life and to maintain OPTIMAL WELLNESS! Therefore, you must continue to do the things necessary in order to keep receiving the benefits!

My Wellness Makeover

When I was 19, in 1991 a woman at my former church, Ozie Holbrook started sharing with me the benefits of taking multi-vitamins, and I have been taking them ever since.

By the time I turned 30; in 2002 I started picking up more weight and ballooned to 185 lbs. and a size 14. I loved food, I still do.

However, I ate just about whatever I wanted. I habitually consumed meat, macaroni and cheese, potatoes, ice cream, chocolate candy, cookies, cakes etc. with just some scant servings of green veggies. I continued to eat the foods that I was accustomed to and assumed that they did no harm.

I then moved to San Diego, then later Los Angeles CA. I went around 3 weeks in San Diego before I saw (1) person who was overweight! I could not believe it!! After I noticed I thought, what's up with that? What are the people here doing? I joined a gym the next week and the gyms were ALWAYS FULL! People on the West Coast, are more health conscious and also want to look good.

In Los Angeles, in 2004 I landed a job with a PR firm and remembered the things my co-worker **Gerson Martinez** from Nordstrom at the Grove shared with me; when I asked how he became so positive & energetic.

He taught me about positive thinking and eating organic foods. The very next day, I spent $100 on organic produce & other organic foods at **Trader Joes!**

At this point I started reading various books about natural foods and other resources which are available to us from Mother Earth. I was astounded to discover all the natural things which are available for our wellness!

With all this good news, I began to question everything that I'd been told by the traditional medical community and the media.

As I was reading the book, I started sharing the good news with my family and friends! Once I cleaned out my own pantry & fridge, I started making calls and suggesting that others do the same! It was how I discovered that refrigerator and pantry makeovers, could be a great step to helping others embrace a new healthy lifestyle!

Did you know the average person can have up to 5-20 pounds of waste in their intestines? How much waste do you have in your gut? What are you willing to do to get it out!!? Also, getting it out and keeping your gut clean, will determine how many nutrients your body is able to assimilate and allow your cells to absorb …to keep maintaining the HEALTHY YOU! To keep my gut clean, clear and to help digest the things I consume; I take digestive enzymes with my meals regularly!

I also do enemas regularly and get colonics occasionally. If you have a dis-ease, are in pain, have low energy, feel depressed etc., embark on a change, start reading more books, attend Holistic fairs, research on-line about natural health. God provided many of the things we need in Nature. Our food, which leads to Wholeness, is our true medicine!

When we use food as our medicine, we can make gradual changes that can become permanent, as our bodies are nourished and healed. Fruit, veggies, nuts, seeds, herbal extracts & essential oils, sea vegetables; they ALL assist the body with repairing itself.

I am so grateful for my friend **Joy Malone,** who taught me about the many benefits of essential oils! As she would put them on me, over a short time I saw a significant change in how I felt spiritually, mentally, emotionally and physically and my hunger for knowledge about them grew and grew! Our ancestors knew how to extract the oils from the plants, fruit & herbs etc., distill them and administer them to people who were ill. They have been around for centuries. Many cultures still have this knowledge and still use them today! Well I'm here to tell you they work!

To hear testimonies about how they have helped people and pets to feel better, visit YouTube.

Services Offered

Would you like to request that I speak to your group about Natural Health? Would you like a single or group, phone or in person Wellness Makeover? I take a look at the foods, beverages, skincare and household products you currently use and make alternative suggestions. Send e-mail to: mskatinalove@gmail.com and your 15 min. phone consultation is free!

"LIKE" my Facebook page here:
www.facebook.com/LotusLifeWellnessCenter

Learn more about the varieties of healthy options which I share through things I post.

My Ongoing Journey

In Awakening To Natural Wellness

In this picture I was at Mackinaw Island. I remember as I prepared for this vacation, I was already mindful of the importance of eating healthy! I knew I would be there a few days, so I planned in advance. I was sure to pack some fruit and nuts for my snacks. Also, I had stopped using the microwave. So instead, I packed my car with a large picnic basket full of goodies, and my new mini toaster oven to heat my food, when warming leftovers from eating out.

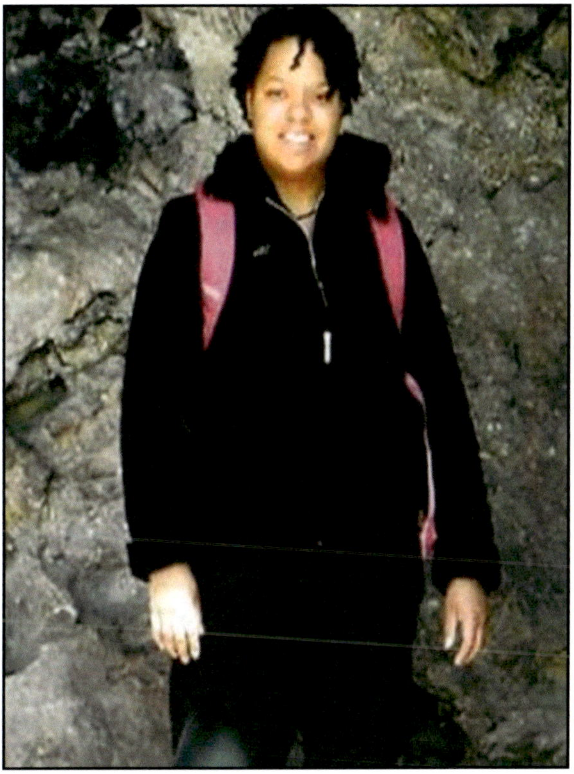

2009 – This is me, looking for change

This is an example of making adjustments to your lifestyle, when it comes to your health. I also had the advantage to go bike riding while visiting Mackinaw Island.

I can remember how exhilarating it felt to embark upon a new way of living! Another light bulb came on for me when I began learning about the importance of consuming raw foods in their *natural state*.

This was realized when I attended a raw food class with Ellen Livingston.

She shared with us how her health shifted when she went on a raw food diet of 80% raw & 20% cooked *...all a plant based diet!*

In this photo, I slenderized my body by consuming mostly raw foods in their natural state ...and taking digestive enzymes. This truly changed my life, and how I now look at food. I feel lighter, sleep better, have more energy, my skin glows, and I feel balanced ...and so much more!

I bought a brand new wardrobe and gave away my old clothes. (Some of which were very nice.) I was glad to, because I had begun a new chapter in my life. Boy, does it feel good to be slender!

There are others I appreciate in my journey, who have taught me what true wellness is, and they are: Dr. Gary Young, Dr. Keefa Loraine Weatherspoon, and Abraham Hicks!

I still consider myself
a student of life,
keeping in mind
that
true wellness
is a
lifelong journey!

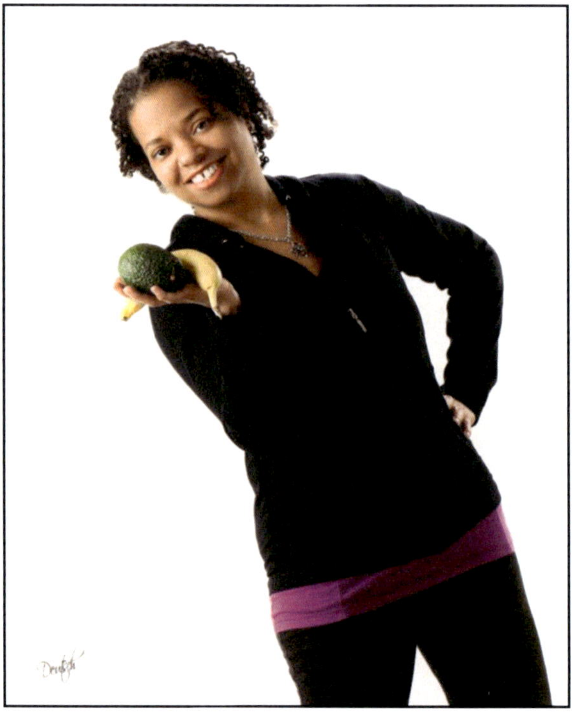

2015 – This is me, Happy and Healthy

A Healthier Lifestyle Begins

It all begins with you. Like everything else in life, if you want to achieve something; you must set the intention to do so first. If your Intention is, to achieve Optimal Health, then start visualizing it now!

Healthy Body Visualization:

Affirmations:

"My Intention is, to remain healthy and discover new things that help me stay on my path."

Or

"My Intention is, to Release all sickness & dis-ease from my body and to become as healthy as I can possibly be".

Visualization

Now take five minutes and visualize yourself on a movie screen in a theatre.

Think of what you want your life to be like... How do you want to feel? Want more Energy? Want to be pain free? Shed Weight? Want to be able to do the things you used to enjoy doing? Want to be healthy in your senior years? Visualize that Now!

You can also tailor your own Affirmations to whatever you desire.

A New Journey

Are you ready to take a journey to consciously improve your life? Start your day off with Gratitude, Prayer & Meditation and then proceed to the following.

Let's look at five quick steps that you can begin with immediately, to start your transformation. They are simple. Dramatic results will begin with the very first step that I am about to share! You can just remember that your action BREWS your new healthy lifestyle. You can "BREW" a whole new you! It is easy! Just change how you:

Breathe,

Rest,

Exercise,

Drink Water,

Enjoy Sunlight.

After we review these first five elements for changing your life, we will discuss diet and lifestyle changes that will dig deeper into the full transformation you have as a goal!

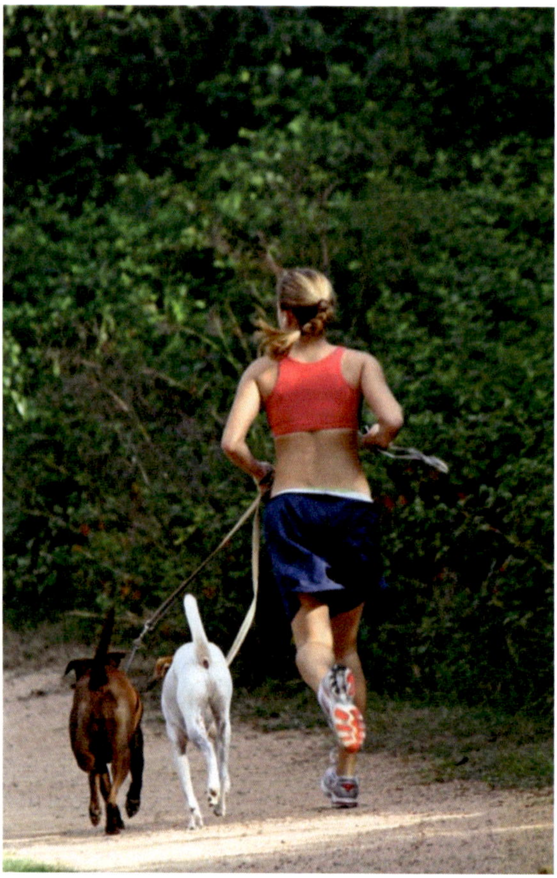

Breathe

Because of breath, we have life. Furthermore, when we start to consciously practice deep breathing, we send oxygen throughout our whole body, including our brain and oxygenating every cell of our being!

We are also improving every area of our health! Getting air to circulate in our environment is also important and we can do that by opening doors and windows in our homes and on rides through the country in our cars.

Plenty of Fresh Air

To maintain optimal health, it is essential to open windows and get fresh air daily! The re-circulated air in office buildings and even some homes can and often does harbor disease. Air quality is important and fresh air infused with the positive energy of being in circulation across the planet does wonders for lifting our mood and improving our health.

Make this your very first step- go ahead- set down this book, and open the window!

Deep Breathing Exercises

Instructions:

1. Inhale: Through your nose, breathe in a long deep breath using your belly to pull the inhalation in. Note: your stomach should expand as you breathe in. I typically count to six as I inhale.

2. Pause: Then hold that inhalation for 3 seconds.

3. Exhale: Then exhale or breathe out of your nose slowly (just as long as it took you to breathe in). Your belly should push down as the air goes out.

For further development, Pranayama yoga emphasizes mastery of many different breathing exercises and studying them can bring a wonderful sense of purification and focus into your life.

I have discovered that deep breathing exercises paired with aroma therapy can be either relaxing or invigorating depending on the oils I use!

Sleep/Rest

Proper Sleep is Essential for Optimal Health. The research on sleep is vast as an internet search will demonstrate. A good night's sleep is essential for physical, spiritual and emotional health. So why are so many people walking around sleep deprived? Insomnia and sleep disorders have increased as we gather our technology around us and find excuses to keep going and "burn the midnight oil."

Dr. Naiman is the author of Healing Night: The Science and Spirit of Sleeping, Dreaming and Awakening.

Take this quiz based on the research in his book. Answer the following questions with a yes or no.

______ How is your sleep health?

______ I can fall asleep the second my head hits the pillow.

______ I usually need to set several alarms to wake me up.

______ I rely on my morning coffee, or the adrenaline rush of running late to appointments or some high glycemic foods to get me through my day.

______ I can't fall asleep without a night-light or TV on in the room.

______ I cannot remember the last dream that I had.

______ I only turn into bed when I can't think of anything else I need to do.

______ I never meditate, pray or try yoga.

If you answered yes to any of the above statements, you are putting your health at risk and setting yourself up for sleep problems. Studies show that a lack of sleep can lead to drowsiness, irritability, and impaired performance of even the simplest tasks and lack of concentration.

According to the Harvard Women's Health Watch, chronic sleep deprivation can be the first source of that weight gain that doesn't want to go away, or even contribute to high blood pressure! When it goes on for an extended period of time, the immune system becomes weakened leading to added health risks. It can also contribute to psychological issues like erratic behavior and mood swings that can become your "new normal." Sleep debt has been linked to tragic incidents such as auto accidents and more.

Remember that the average adult requires six to eight hours of restful deep sleep. During sleep there are cycles of REM (rapid eye movements and Non-Rem sleep. When you get past the first four hours, you enter into a REM cycle and have dreams, which are deeply beneficial. Sleep helps the brain to commit information to memory via memory consolidation. In a way, our brains get a nice workout while our bodies are inactive and healing during sleep. Foods and beverages we consume do affect our quality of sleep. Choose wisely and your body will thank you!

This is why it is best to finish your last meal of the day, at least 3-5 hours before bedtime. If you must consume something in the later part of evening or night, you could drink 2-4 ounces of your chosen alternative, non-dairy milk and add powered Spirulina or Cinnamon (optional).

Enhance the quality of your sleep

Ideally, with the perfect conditions, it would be a good practice to turn off all electronics such as: televisions, cellular phones, alarm clocks, cd players, computers, laptops, notepads, iPods, video games, and electric heaters. Never sleep with electric blankets!

Should you require leaving your cell phone or home phone on, you can either put it outside the room you sleep in or position it at the far end of the room, from where you sleep; being at least 10 feet away from where you sleep.

Also, sleep with room dark, light and the above mentioned, can disrupt sleep pattern, heart rhythm and nervous system.

"Me Time" just before bed

What you do before you sleep are the thoughts you take with you into your rest! Reading a spiritually uplifting/self-help book or listening to spiritual/ inspirational music will also help you to drift off to a good night's rest. In addition, take the time to recite positive affirmations and or prayers. Be diligent and insure that nothing or no one serves as distractions for this, including telephone ringing, television on in the background or other interferences.

Affirmation: I am taking time out for myself and becoming healthier & healthier.

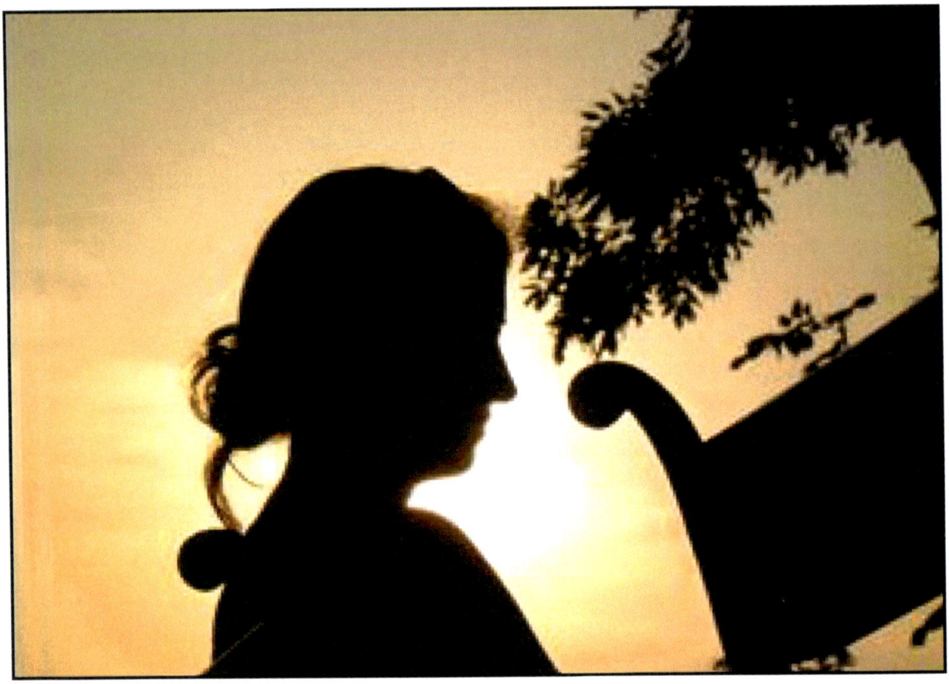

Great Sleep Aides

When I experienced a serious bout of insomnia, Essential Oil Therapy helped me. There are several ways that essential oils can be used:

- Waft the scent under your nostrils while deep breathing.
- Take a warm steamy bath with several drops mixed in.
- Massage a drop or two into your wrists and throat
- Add a few drops on your pillow
- Use a diffuser to move it through the bedroom.

I use Lavender and Cedar wood essential oils or "sleep essence," which comes in a capsule and contains a soothing mixture of five essential oils including Valerian and Lavender.

Exercise

Our bodies were designed to move and be active. This is without question. Be sure to get proper exercise daily. The best value that comes from a program of regular exercise: it causes your body to release Serotonin and Endorphins, known as the happy hormones.

Recommended Exercises

Proceed at your own discretion

Daily morning stretches is a great way to use muscles that may not otherwise be used on a regular basis. The following is a great guide, to stretch and feel the benefits!

It's recommended to stretch before any exercise. Stretching is the best way to reduce injury. There are numerous videos on YouTube you can check out on how to stretch before working out.

Want to make Yoga part of your daily routine?

Invest in an Eco-friendly yoga mat and yoga mat carrier to keep it clean when traveling: Buy on-line, **Whole Foods** or **TJ Maxx** may carry.

Walking or other cardio activities (30 min.-1 hour) 4 times per week are great ways to get your weekly exercise in. Below are more creative ways to work out!

Creative ways to work out:

- Zumba Workout
- Your favorite cardio DVD
- Bike Riding
- Salsa or Ballroom Dancing
- Yoga
- Hiking
- Beach Body DVD set
- Classes at your local gym
- Dancing to YouTube music
- Mountain climbing
- Swimming
- Taking the stairs instead
- Parking as far away from the door when shopping, visiting, etc.

Improve your vision

Exercise to improve eye health: Look up and down, side-to- side (repeat) Benefits: keep eyes toned and strong. Also if you use a computer regularly, step away from it every hour or so, and give your eyes a break between your projects, as using the computer screen can cause vision stress.

Water

Drink plenty of Alkaline Water

Staying hydrated is so very important! Pure water is a key element in being well & is vital for life. Alkaline water has been proven to help balance the PH in the human body and its molecules are small enough to penetrate cells in the human body; so they can provide the body with the proper hydration that it needs and increase energy level! The average person may want to drink ½ their body weight in ounces each day.

Sunlight

Sunlight is essential to life!! It radiates energy to our planet and all inhabitants on it! Remember: you want to get in-tuned with you, listen to your intuition & your body. You will begin to know what lengths of time in the sun are right for you; regardless of what others may say about it! I personally love the sun and get sunlight as much as possible! Also keep in mind; we still need sunlight during winter months! I make sure I consistently take vitamin D and calcium supplements especially during this time, especially if I am in a colder climate!

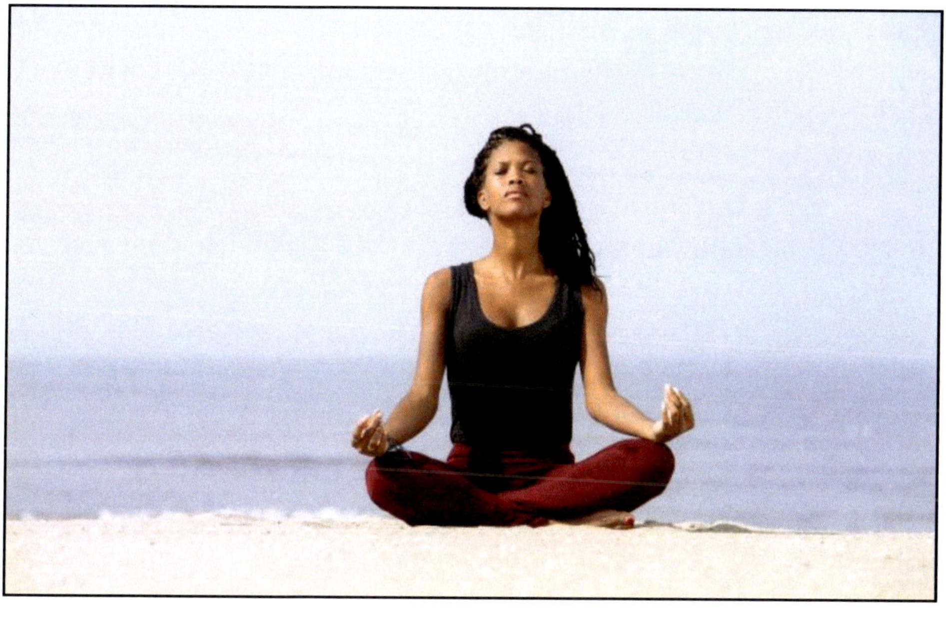

Music Therapy: Sound

This also reminds me of the Power of Sound! Sound Creates, Uplifts and Heals! When I think of Sound, I think about the Creator, how the world came into form with all the inhabitants! Sound Creates Life & Vitality!!

Relaxation and Stress Reduction

If you like or are open to Meditation, Yoga and Spiritual music, this may be a good website for you. The music from this website has truly been a blessing to me over the years! www.soundstrue.com/store

Keep in mind, music should always be Positive and Uplifting! The lyrics of music make a huge difference. The idea is to use music to improve your mood and your life. Always choose music with Positive lyrics and instrumental is just as good!

Time can always be set aside, to enjoy your favorite music! While getting dressed in the morning, while preparing food, doing chores, in the car or during me time etc.

There are so many benefits to Positive music. Music heals, soothes, uplifts and can put you in a Positive mindset! If you want to get started with a good day, play some music! Many successful business people and those who just want to be happy, use motivational music to get them started each morning. It's an excellent motivator!

Help with Memory

I saw the video of an elderly man who had Alzheimers. He had been depressed for years and did not remember much. His therapist played his favorite song from his era and he became alive again! The moment he could hear the music, his face lit up and he started singing! He could also remember every word! This was an amazing analysis and shows the Positive effect music can have on us!

To watch the video, go to YouTube and type:
(Original) Man in Nursing Home reacts to hearing music from his era

Get more info about improving memory here!
www.musicandmemory.org

So know that what you choose makes the BREWS you use!

B is for ____________________ because it

____

R is for ____________________ important because

____

E is for ____________________ which releases

____________________ happy chemicals.

W is for ____________________ the best type for

full use is ____________________________________

S is for ____________________ as it is our main

source of ______________________________________

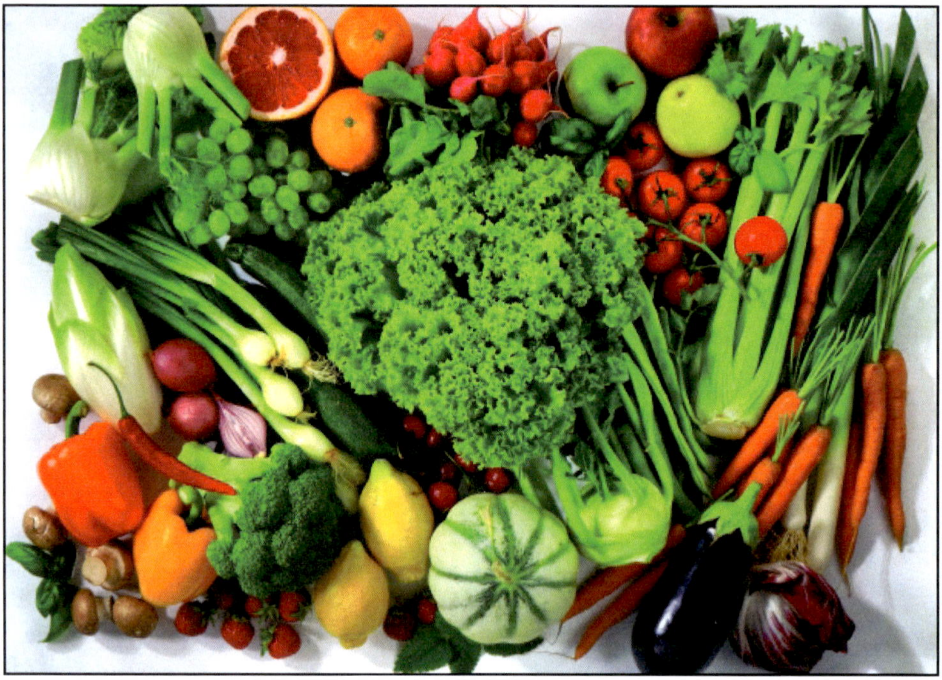

Suggestions On What To Consume

(Diet and Nutrition Changes)

Consider a diet of 50% raw foods

Your body is always working, doing its best to keep you alive and as well as possible. Your part is to feed it authentic substances (real foods) to allow this process to take place.

All of all bodies are different, what works for one person may not work for another. The following are suggestions of the type of foods that may be beneficial for certain blood types. You may want to do further research on your blood type and diet that is best for you. If this resonates with you, here's a great place to start: **www.dadamo.com**

The three basic things to remember about changing your diet:

FIRST, Start when and how you can. Some will be able to implement every change immediately.

I do offer pantry and refrigerator makeovers to make this possible. I can do phone or internet consultations or travel to your site if you prefer.

If you are going to start gradually, try changing either one meal each day. This can be done by incorporating dark leafy greens or spring mix (salad) and more veggies.

"The base of my diet is green, green foods give life, especially raw leafy greens"!

SECOND, Adapt to new information and research, by becoming a student of nutrition. Did you know that your typical physician takes less than four hours' worth of nutritional training? This is why so many doctors typically treat symptoms with medications and assume that everything can be remedied with pain relievers and pills.

THIRD, you can make better choices and do it affordably and with pleasure if you remember why you are doing this! Foods, which are in their whole and unprocessed form, are always the best choice. Whenever possible, foods should be eaten this way. Think **RAWER!** Raw greens, veggies, roots, (some steamed/cooked), seeded fruit, nuts, etc.

Organic Foods

These are foods that are produced using methods of organic farming – ones that do not involve modern synthetic inputs such as, synthetic pesticides and chemical fertilizers.

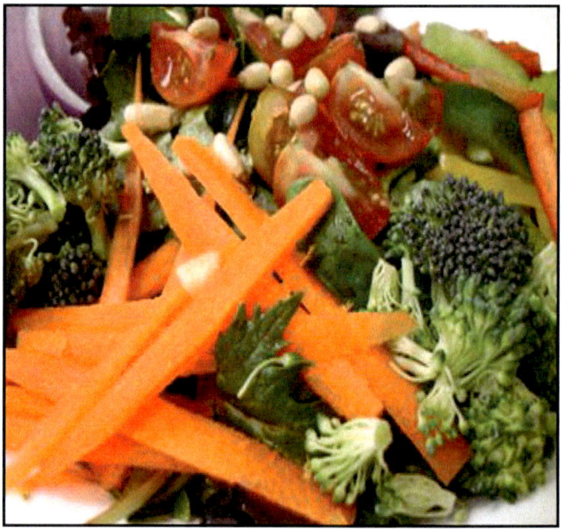

Organic foods are also not processed using irradiation, industrial solvents, or chemical food additives, in any form.

I recommend a simple and easy to manage diet. Buy Organic whenever possible and from local farmers and growers, starting with the Farmer's Market. As the basis, this can consist of a combination of the following: Fresh, raw organic leafy greens, raw fruit, raw sprouted and cooked veggies, sprouted and cooked beans, sprouted and cooked lentils, certain sprouted and cooked grains and raw nuts, seeds, sea vegetables and seaweeds. When seeds are soaked and dehydrated, this allows for the best digestion and nutrient absorption.

Leafy Greens, Veggies and Fruit

The base of my diet is green and this is a mixture of the following: Raw Organic dark leafy greens, parsley, chard, kale, cilantro & other green herbs. The liquid compounds inside the plants are identical to the human blood plasma. When we consume greens in their raw natural state, we get the full benefits of them. There are many essential nutrients present in leafy greens, veggies and brightly colored fruit as well! My experience has been, to eat as much Raw, Organic dark leafy greens, fruit and veggies as possible! Eating a wide variety of the color spectrum in dark leafy greens, fruit and veggies can help you to meet your nutritional needs and boost your Energy Level! Add as much color and variety to your plate as possible!

For weight and carbohydrate reduction: enjoy a sweet potato or yam instead of white or red skin potatoes. Enjoy the natural taste with a sprinkle of the Pink Himalayan Salt and or cinnamon; don't overload it with any fancy toppings, which can mask the flavor.

FYI: Avocados are especially good for strengthening the reproductive system for both men and women.

Fruit Seeds

Fruit seeds are invaluable because they have many vital minerals in them. Think about this, anything with a seed inside of it is considered a fruit and many of them are edible!

Such as: honeydews, cantaloupes, squash, and many more! When opening these to eat, instead of throwing out the seeds scoop them out and blend them in your blender! The nutrients inside of them are invaluable. I even eat watermelon and grapefruit seeds. If you do eat seeds from fruit however, they must be chewed really well in order for the body to break down the nutrients.

Super Foods

Super foods are foods which are nutrient-rich and excellent for health and well-being! Some of which include: berries, chlorella, spirulina, chia seeds, quinoa, broccoli, sweet potatoes, dark leafy greens, pomegranate, watermelon, nuts, seeds, cocoa, salmon and many more!

Antioxidants

Antioxidants are a vital part of our diet. These help to protect our bodies of free radicals that can enter through breathing toxic substances and foreign particles, such as: dust, mold, residue from toxic chemicals in the home or office and outdoor pollutants. Several sources include fruits, veggies, organic apple cider vinegar, herbs, spices, teas, and you can add **Genesis Today** noni, mangosteen and Acai berry juices as well as therapeutic essential oils, which can be applied topically, and some can be ingested.

Protein

Protein is necessary for the proper building and functioning of the human body. Many people have been conditioned to think we need to consume enormous amounts from fish, poultry or meat. My experience has been that we may not need as much as we have been lead to believe. Get in tuned with and listen to your body. You will intuitively start to know how much is required for you as an individual. Your overall level of activity is a huge determining factor of how much protein you may need.

Natural Sources of Protein

These include raw/organic leafy greens including kale, chard, mustard, collard greens, bean sprouts, broccoli sprouts, spirulina powder, wheat grass, raw nuts and seeds. I also recommend slow cooked beans and lentils, consumed in moderation. All these help to meet daily protein requirements.

Sprouted Vegetables, Seeds, Lentils and Beans

When you eat sprouted foods instead of cooked, you get the maximum amount of absorption and assimilation of nutrients, enzymes and more flavor! You can find these at Whole Foods Market, your local health food store or prepare your own!

Ann Wigmore, a pioneer in Natural Health, has a book '***Recipes for Longer Life***' with lots of information and recipes on how to sprout. I had a field day exploring all the great ideas she shared in her book and grateful for her knowledge she left for us! Order on Amazon!

Beans, Legumes and Lentils (slow cooked)

Both beans and lentils contain protein, vitamins, minerals and fiber and can be good for your overall health. Some of which, are complete sources of protein, which means they contain all 9 required amino acids, to support proper body function.

How to Prepare Beans:

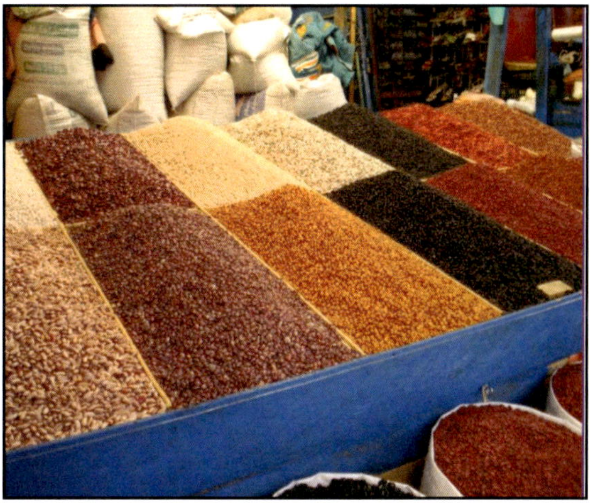

I recommend that you pre-soak them 6 to 8 hours before cooking, using a large glass jar, ceramic or stainless steel cooking dish. This reduces the cooking time and possibly preserves more nutrients. If room temperature is cool, leave out; if not then store in fridge. Be sure to leave lid loose, so that gasses can escape and the jar does not burst. Before cooking, you must rinse them well. Cook on low temperature for an extended time. I recommend using a slow cooker.

Whole Grains

Grains should be a selective choice. My recommendation is to choose grains that are easy to digest such as, amaranth, millet and teff. Quinoa is classified as a grain but, actually is a seed. This is another option also.

Meat, Fish and Poultry

Meat, fish and poultry should always be eaten in moderation. My experience has been, consuming large amounts of meat, fish or poultry can be stressful on the digestive system and can take huge amounts of energy to properly digest! These items become more optional, for many who are discovering and embracing a diet with more raw and plant based foods. For the average person, when eating these remember the size to consider is a serving which fits into the palm of your hand. I also will split a portion into 2 meals. Eating this three to four times per week for me is sufficient. When I do consume these, I also increase my activity level to reflect the added calories, fat and to help with digestion which is essential! If you would like to exercise and can't, start to visualize yourself being more active! This may take some getting used to if you are used to consuming large portions of meat; perhaps you can incorporate more beans & vegetables into your diet, along with the smaller portion sizes of meat.

It's recommended for everyone to explore and experiment with different foods, to find out what works best for you.

Again, find out your blood type; then research the types of foods that may suit you.

How to select Animal proteins

If you choose to eat red meats, chicken, or poultry purchase your products from a local Farmer's Market whenever possible.

Take a moment to actually talk with the farmer and insure that they operate from a place of integrity! Find out if their animals are fed Non-GMO grains, such as organic soybeans or are grass fed. Beef should always be grass fed and can be found at some farmer's markets or meat specialty shops. It is worth the price and effort to find quality red meats. If they use corn as their feed, it may be GMO or of a lesser quality.

Also, it's best when the animals are treated with respect and compassion before it becomes part of a meal. If this interests you, I highly recommend reading works from autistic researcher and animal behaviorist Temple Grandin, PhD.

When shopping for fish, always choose fish, which still has the fins and scales. I recommend you choose a fishery that catches its fish direct from oceans and lakes that are low in mercury and other toxins. Also, buy fish that does not have color or other preservatives added. As a chain store, I consider Whole Foods Market to be a good source.

Essential Fatty Acids Omega-3-6-9s

These are critical for the body. From joint health to skin and circulation, oils are often underappreciated for what they add to our bodies. Be sure to rotate nuts, seeds and oils from time to time.

Omega-3

My favorite sources include raw walnuts, un-refined walnut oil, hemp seeds, flaxseed and un-refined flaxseed oil.

Omega-6

An important nutrient for proper heart function; Omega-6 may reduce the risk of heart disease. Sources I recommend include nuts and seeds such as pistachios, pecans, Brazil nuts and sunflower seeds. Another great way is to add flax or sesame seed oils to your food once prepared and cooked; or cooking with sesame seed oils on low-medium heat.

Omega-9

Good sources for Omega-9 are found in unrefined olive and sunflower oils. These oils are best when poured on top of food after cooking. It is important to know that cooking with olive oils or sunflower oils, causes a change in its chemistry, and can produce substances that may be harmful to the human body.

Suggested Cooking Oils

I strongly recommend **Spectrum** Organic Unrefined Virgin Coconut or Unrefined Sesame Seed oil. This can be readily purchased at your local health food store.

Good Fats

We need and use fats (or lipids) for energy and energy storage. They also play an important role in proper functioning of the body and help to protect our organs. The challenge is that we can consume the wrong types of fats and more than we require if we don't watch ourselves.

Excellent sources I recommend include: avocados, olives, pecans, walnuts, hazelnuts, cashews, pine nuts etc. These food sources eaten in moderation generally do not cause weight gain. Other places to find good fats include coconut, olive, walnut oil, and avocado oils. Read the labels and be sure to only choose unrefined oils. When choosing olive oil, I recommend that you specifically choose only Organic and Extra Virgin.

Alternative, Healthy Beverages

Drinking fresh, young coconut water, herbal and fruit teas can be a healthy alternative to other beverages. I have found that making the choice to eliminate all processed drinks such as soda pop, artificial fruit juices and more is critical to achieving your health and wellness goals. Even the ones you drank growing up!!

Fresh Young Coconut Water

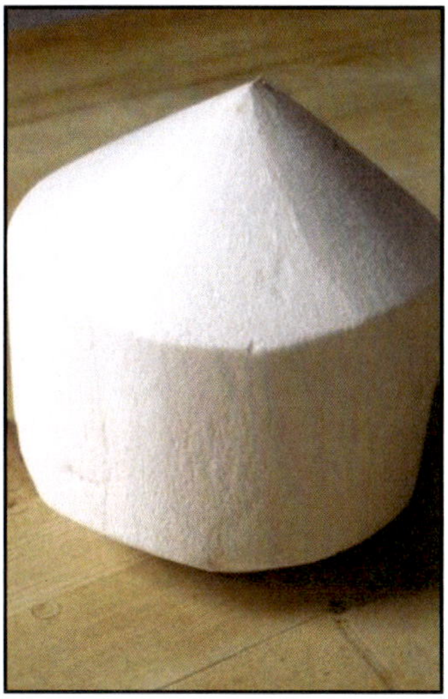

Fresh young white Thai coconut water has been in the media of late and for good reasons. It contains the same amount of electrolytes as the human plasma and can be a lifesaver! If I share nothing else with you, I want you to know that fresh, young coconut water is my absolute favorite beverage on the planet! The mature coconut is also nutritious; however I choose young white Thai whenever possible!

In 2010, I had a physical and my blood drawn (6 tubes) to check my mineral levels. This appointment came during a time I had been fasting. Looking back, it would have been better to postpone my appointment. However, the next day I woke up feeling really weak and proceeded to run errands anyway.

While driving, I became very lightheaded and chose to drive to Whole Foods Market *(praying the whole time)*. I went straight to the produce department and picked up a fresh young coconut. I asked the produce associate to open it for me. He did. I proceeded to drink the entire 8 ounces right inside the grocery store. Immediately, I started feeling my energy level restored! I sincerely believe this choice to drink the fresh, young coconut water saved me from passing out or ultimately saved my life!

Tea

Herbal and fruit teas can have many positive benefits on health. These contain antioxidants, vitamins, minerals and have been around for thousands of years.

Best tea to purchase: whenever possible, consume loose tea. They can be purchased at your local health food store or Whole Foods at a reasonable price, in the bulk foods section. My personal recommendation for drinking tea: herbal or fruit loose tea, muslin drawstring tea bags. I prefer using thick ceramic mugs/coffee mugs.

Some of my favorite varieties include Nettles, Peppermint, Rooibos, Par de Arco, and Blueberry. Herbal teas are loaded with nutrients!

Tea can be enjoyed at room temperature to best preserve the nutrients. However, herbal tea should be heated up to temperature, but should not ever boil. This myth comes from the sound of the singing tea kettle. Never heat the loose tea leaves themselves; instead the water should be slightly heated to about 'bath water warm.'

How to prepare for drinking as a 'cold' beverage: pour alkaline or purified water in glass jar with lid. Add dry tea to a muslin tea bag, and then steep inside water for 30 minutes. Enjoy!

You can save and store your tea bag in another jar with lid and use again for another serving. Be sure to store this in refrigerator.

Research has shown when a tea bag is immersed in room temperature Alkaline Water; it steeps in the same as it would in hot water with all the colors released into the water.

Note: *some herbal teas such as from bark or root may require heating to release all of the nutritive properties.*

If you are a strong coffee drinker thinking of embracing more tea into your life, the more tea you immerse into your water, the stronger it is. I personally like my tea strong! An added benefit to this is a bonus to your health!

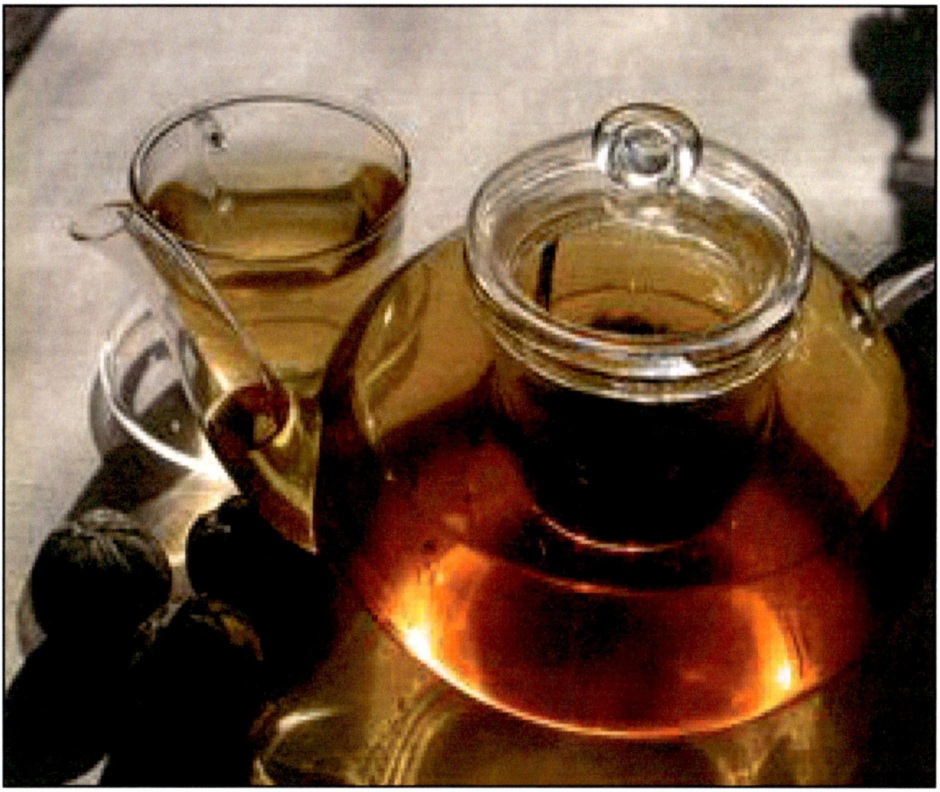

Tips For Grocery Shopping

Think More Fresh Foods And Preparing From Scratch!

Keep in mind when shopping; there may be many things available that you may not have tried before. Be open to trying new things like, exotic fruit. If you are not sure of what it is, get the name of it and explore on-line before purchasing. I try new things all the time and I am always excited when grocery shopping, to see what new fruit or veggie I can try. Also, when shopping for fruit, vegetables and produce, keep the following in mind:

- Have something to eat before shopping, to be sure You buy what You need to stay within your budget
- Select produce that looks the freshest
- Buy organic as much as possible
- Items that go by the weight may have excess water on them, be sure to shake off as much as possible
- Never buy apples that look shiny (they are coated with wax)
- Some stores sell dark leafy greens by the weight, this may be a better price
- Use the least amount of plastic bags as possible
- Re-use your own bags for overall grocery shopping
- Monitor what goes on sale regularly
- Get to know produce dept. associate & days items come in
- You may place special orders for certain items ahead of time
- Inform the store manager if you do not see an item you'd like store to carry

SNAP

Some people are not aware that those who have EBT cards can purchase powder and liquid supplements. For example: powdered Spirulina and liquid Noni juice, if supplement is in this form it can be purchased this way.

If you are diabetic, when shopping for fruit it is recommended that you are mindful with your selections and eat fruit in moderation. Do your own research, talk to your health practitioner and always listen to your body!

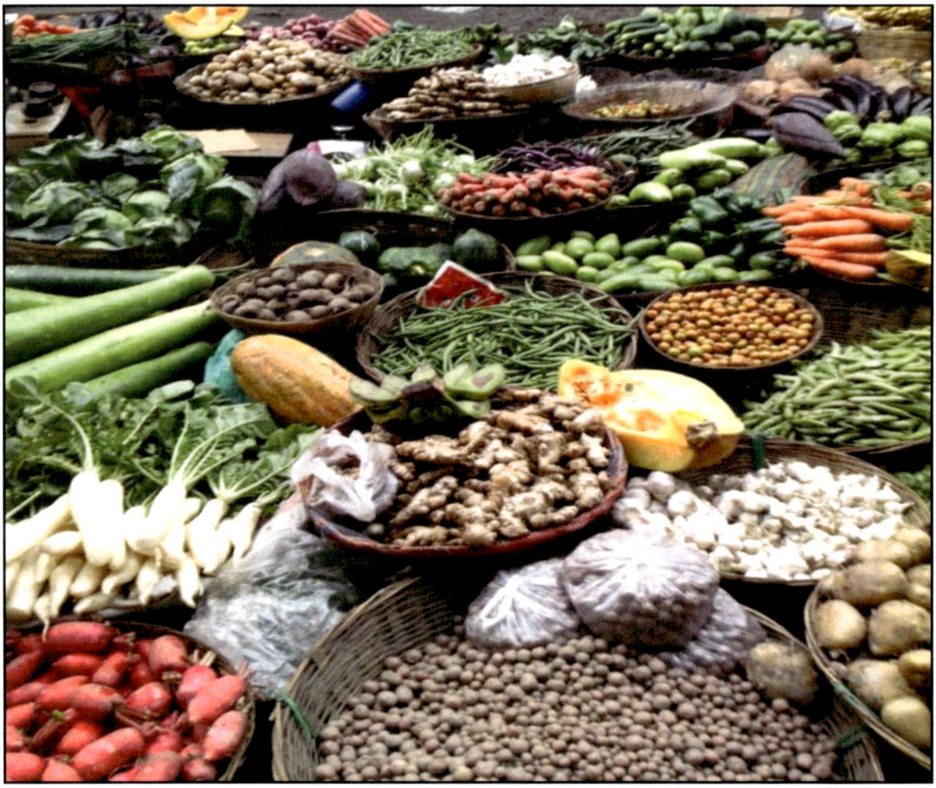

STARTER HEALTHY GROCERY LIST

Fruit

- Bananas
- Mangos
- Blue Berries
- Strawberries
- Grapefruit
- Oranges
- Tangerines
- Cantaloupe
- Avocado
- Watermelon

More of what you like

Vegetables Raw fresh or frozen

- Squash
- Green beans
- Organic Salad-Mixed Greens
- Green, Red and Yellow Peppers
- Onions
- Garlic
- Sweet Potatoes
- Mixed Veggies
- Sprouts *(Raw)*
- Adzuki bean sprouts
- Alfalfa sprouts
- Mixed bean sprouts
- Broccoli sprouts
- Green lentil sprouts

Whole Grains

- Quinoa
- Teff
- Kamut
- Amaranth
- Millet

Superfood Powders

- Beet powder
- Acai Berry
- Spirulina

Nuts and Seeds (*Raw is best)*

- Brazil nuts
- Walnuts
- Macadamia nuts
- Cashews
- Pecans
- Pistachios (unsalted)
- Hazelnuts
- Almonds
- Pine nuts
- Sunflower seeds
- Pumpkin seeds

Healthy Oils

(*Rotate and always choose un-refined***)**

- Coconut Oil (*Best for cooking*)
- Sesame Seeds Oil
- Grapeseed Oil

Legumes (Raw and dry, canned not recommended)

- Adzuki beans
- Lima beans
- Green, brown and red lentils
- Chick pea or garbanzo beans
- Fava beans

Bread

- (*Best if avoided, if you must)* Ezekiel bread (health food stores)

Super fruit Juices

- *Genesis Today Brand*
- Resveratrol
- Noni
- Mangosteen
- Acai Berry
- Seaweeds
- Nori
- Kelp
- Dulse
- Wakame

Proteins

- Fish with fins and scales (without color added)
- Free range chicken (*without color added*)

Nut butters

- Spices & Seasonings
- Almond butter
- Cinnamon
- Cashew butter
- Clove

Condiments

- Nutmeg
- Bragg apple cider vinegar
- Ginger
- Fresh lemon or lime
- Garlic powder
- Liquid aminos spray (contains soy)
- Paprika (Contains soy)
- Curry
- Vinaigrette salad dressings
- Cilantro

How To Store Fruit, Veggies and Leafy Greens

Always store salads & dark leafy greens in the fridge

Store bananas outside of fridge

When temperature is neutral to cool inside your home, you may store potatoes, onions & garlic outside of fridge, otherwise store inside fridge

Fruit & veggies you plan to eat in next 1-3 days may be safe to store outside of fridge depending on their ripeness

Preparing your own meals

I strongly recommend it's best to prepare for these new ways of eating in advance. Always have a plan for each meal ready ahead of time, before you get hungry. You have a much better chance of eating more healthy foods. If you are busy working or on the go, prepare at night or in the morning and your food packed in proper container(s), so that you can grab and go! There are thermal lunch bags available in a variety of colors at **Target** and **T.J. Maxx.**

It's also important to have a timer in your kitchen, especially if you are a multi-tasker. This helps to make sure your foods turn out just the way you want them.

Sample Healthy Diet Plan:

(Use your own discretion or consult with your doctor before changing your diet)

Keep in mind, ideally most people sleep at night, which is when your body rests, repairs itself and fasts. Therefore the first meal of the day in the morning can be a light one; and may include but not limited to the following:

Breakfast: the following can be consumed over the course of your morning

First, drink a glass (4-16 oz. or more) of alkaline water first thing in the morning

- Herbal, kombucha or fruit tea of your choice (optional)
- Whole organic, raw fruit
- Fruit Smoothie with or w/o organic leafy greens or Vegetable Juice (can alternate)

See below for recipes

(Optional) add to smoothies Garden of Eden, Meal Replacement or Protein Shake from your health food store.

Lunch and Dinner:

First, drink a glass (4-16 oz. or more) of Alkaline water 30 min before meal

- Spring Mix Salad, Herbal Spring Mix, Romaine Lettuce (Organic) (alternate)
- Shredded carrots
- Red-Yellow–Orange, Green peppers (alternate)
- Olive-Walnut or Sesame seed oil on top (alternate)
- Garbanzo, kidney, navy or pinto beans or green lentils (alternate)
- Sweet Potato (on occasion)
- Quinoa, Millet, wild or black rice (alternate)
- Hummus (optional)
- Mixed Nuts (eat in moderation)
- Small-medium portions of meat, fish or poultry a few times per week.
- During off times, substitute with beans or lentils
- Variety of vegetables such as: broccoli, cauliflower, eggplant, carrots, red cabbage etc.

Snack ideas:

- Apples, oranges or your favorite fruit
- Watermelon
- Fruit Smoothies
- Sorbet (without added sugar)
- Hand full of berries
- Hand full of dried fruit (avoid if yeast/Candida is present)
- Celery, carrots and cauliflower
- Snap pea chips Whole Foods, (Wal-Mart in produce area) or
- Inner Pea's (Trader Joe's)
- Dipped in hummus or salsa
- Variety of nuts (handful)
- Coconut shreds (can toast in 5-10min on stovetop) Also good on salads
- Green peas

Consume in place of snack:

- Herbal or fruit tea
- Young coconut water (fresh from young or mature coconut (white or brown)
- Almond, hemp, or rice milk with small amount of Cinnamon and Clove or Spirulina

**Can also be a late night beverage if dinner is skipped.*

Sweets:

If you choose to still buy and consume store bought ice cream, pies, cookies and cakes; get familiar with reading ingredient labels and buy ones with the most natural ingredients possible.

Ice cream alternatives

- Fruit Smoothies or sorbet
- Homemade ice cream Find recipes on YouTube.

Yummy Recipes

Smoothie Recipes--Great for Breakfast or Snack!

2-4 bananas, cup of blueberries or mixed berries, almond, hemp or rice milk.

2-4 bananas, Mixed Greens: kale, chard, mustard or collard greens (rotate) almond, hemp, or rice milk and ice

Raw Coconut Soup or Pudding

You will need 3-5 Young Thai Coconuts (Purchase at Kroger, Whole Foods Market or your local Health Food Store!)

- 24 oz. Coconut Water
- 4 cups Coconut Meat
- 2 oz. Raw Organic Ginger
- ¼ tsp. Curry or Turmeric
- ¼ tsp Ginger Powder
- Pinch of Salt *(Pink Himalayan or Sea Salt)*
- Organic Ginger Root
- Curry or Turmeric
- Ginger Powder

Bean/Lentil, Vegetable and Quinoa Salad

- Start with your favorite beans or lentils
- Season with: ginger, garlic powder, thyme, cayenne pepper, Himalayan Salt
- Cook quinoa on low heat 15-20 minutes (*for best results, pre-soak 2-4 hours in fridge, before cooking)*
- Steam green peas and mixed veggies for short time
- Add onions and red peppers (if desired) 5-min or so before stovetop is turned off
- Add raw mixed greens and unrefined toasted sesame seed or olive oil

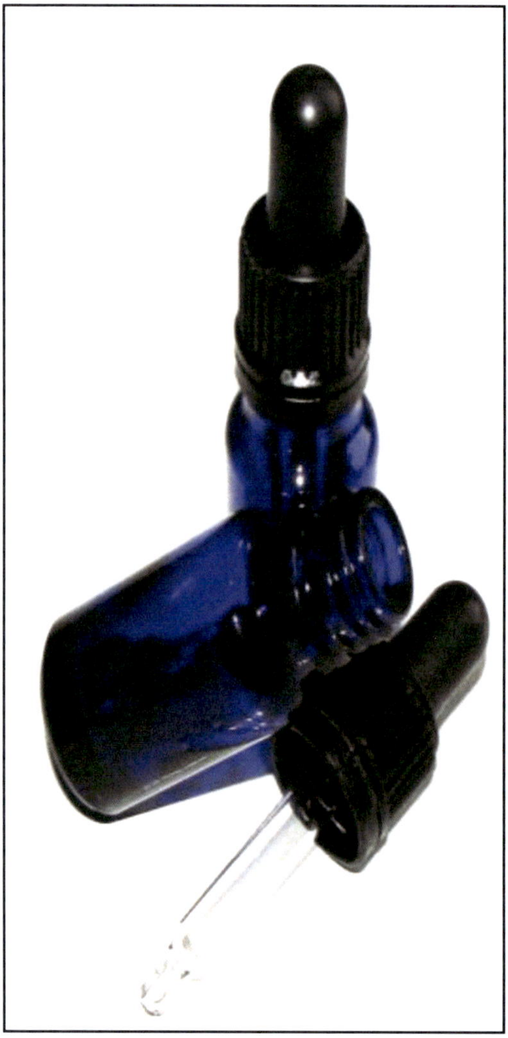

Important Supplements

Essential Oils

There are essential oils available to us from the Garden of Eden; that are extracted from flowers, herbs, trees and shrubs to enhance your spiritual, emotional, mental and physical well-being. These essential oils have played a tremendous role in the improvement in my health!

My personal testimonial

I got relief from a Thyroid imbalance, while working in an environment which did lots of printing with toner. After 2 months of symptoms with missed menstrual cycle and not so easy bowel movements complications; I used Valor essential oil and all symptoms went away in 2 weeks! My period came back and bowel movements were regular again (2-3per day)!

I recommend that you go to YouTube and research "**Benefits of therapeutic grade essential oils.**"

Multi-vitamins

I strongly recommend New Chapter, which is Whole Foods plant based supplement. It is specifically designed for Women's Health and Men's Health.

Calcium

Algae-cal capsules I have found to be an outstanding source. You can order directly from **www.algaecal.com** or can purchase **New Chapter**-Bone Heath tablets from Whole Foods or your local health food store. Ask if they have coupons for you on site!

Vitamin D

My suggestion: **Now Brand** produces Vitamin D, which is lanolin derived from sheep's wool and comes in small gel capsules; it is also very affordable!

Magnesium & Trace Minerals

Magnesium is an important electrolyte and is vital for life and may not be in sufficient amounts in the SAD (Standard American Diet). Therefore it is highly recommended to take as a supplement, as I do daily in 2 ways.

Derma Mag is a magnesium spray with other trace minerals and I spray on bottom of my feet at night before bedtime. I am also sure to take beforehand, my second dose of AlgaeCal or Bone Strength, which is a calcium supplement; with my last meal of the day. This ensures my body is balanced with the proper mixture of minerals that it requires to work at optimal level.

Concen Trace liquid minerals has over 72 trace minerals and is a good source for a high level of magnesium also. They can be consumed with water.

I have both of the above mentioned on-hand at all times, so that I am sure I get sufficient amounts of this vital mineral magnesium! It is important here to read the labels on both, to make sure you are getting sufficient amounts daily.

As benefits of taking in the magnesium supplements, one may experience a better sleep and easier bowel movements.

Enzymes

There are many types of enzymes necessary for healthy living. Digestive Enzymes make it possible for our bodies to break down and assimilate the foods we eat in order to get the maximum amount of nutrition from our foods. My experience has shown that a diet rich in enzymes can increase your energy and stamina, as well as support shedding weight, healthy skin, and overall good health.

When we cook our foods, we destroy the vital enzymes inside them. This is one reason why it's so important to eat raw vegetables such as a healthy salad before cooked foods. I have found that if I have an apple 30 minutes before I have a meal, this will make me feel fuller and I actually eat less.

Each time I consume a meal with cooked foods, I make an effort to eat raw foods before or with them! My experience has shown me time and time again that it is ideal to eat at least 50% of the food I consume daily, raw.

Taking **Enzymedica's** digestive enzymes, **Digest Gold** before meals with cooked foods also make a huge difference! This particular formula may be an excellent choice for people who need extra help with digesting fats, cooked foods and those who do not have a gall bladder. **Enzymedica** carries an array of digestive enzymes depending on the particular needs for your body.

Probiotics

Your intestinal tract is designed to support lots of friendly bacteria, which play an important role in digestion, absorption of nutrients, immunity and disease prevention. Probiotic foods contain living organisms which can complement the bacteria alive in your gut already. With our modern day lifestyle, most peoples' bodies do not produce enough of these friendly bacteria. Foods that contain probiotics are proven to boost immunity, energy levels and overall well-being.

They may also be helpful to those who have issues with their bowels, lung infections, vaginal infections, skin disorders, colds and more!

Some fruits and vegetables have them in small amounts.

I recommend the supplement **Live 5 probiotics** which is very effective and can be ordered on the above website. **Jarrow Brand** probiotics is another great choice and is available at **Whole Foods Market.**

A great probiotic Beverage is **Kombucha.** This comes in many assorted flavors. Whenever I feel like a cold or sniffle may come on, I am sure to grab one or a few of these!!

The young man who founded the company GT'S produces unique blends of a **Kombucha** beverage. He has an awesome story about what drove him to distribute these miraculous drink blends. Once you know it, you too will feel Inspired!

Note:

If you purchase the product, you may want to start out with a small amount first because it's a very powerful beverage!

Find out all the details at: **www.synergydrinks.com**

Release From Lifestyle

Right now, commit to becoming one of the world's greatest readers of food labels.

This is crucial for the changes you want to make and detecting the ingredients in food you want to avoid. Shop when you have time to look at both the ingredient panel and the nutrition fact listings.

You see the words "Fat-free," "Reduced Fat," "Sugar-free" and more on the packaging. If the label says "Free," this doesn't necessarily mean you are free from harm. If the label reads any of these, it has to be replaced with something else. More often than not, that replacement product could be just as harmful.

It has been my experience that real and healthy foods sometimes contain fats. These can be good fats and generally will not cause weight gain. The key is eating in moderation. Avocados and nuts both contain high amounts of fats. I eat these almost daily and still maintain a healthy weight. However, there are fats to be concerned about. Pay attention to fats from meat, fish, poultry, all animal products and artificial fats, which are not from real foods. For optimal health and maintenance of a healthy weight, steer clear of gluten and bread products.

Stop Smoking

If you are a smoker, nothing else you can do will add quality and years to your life like stopping cigarette smoking.

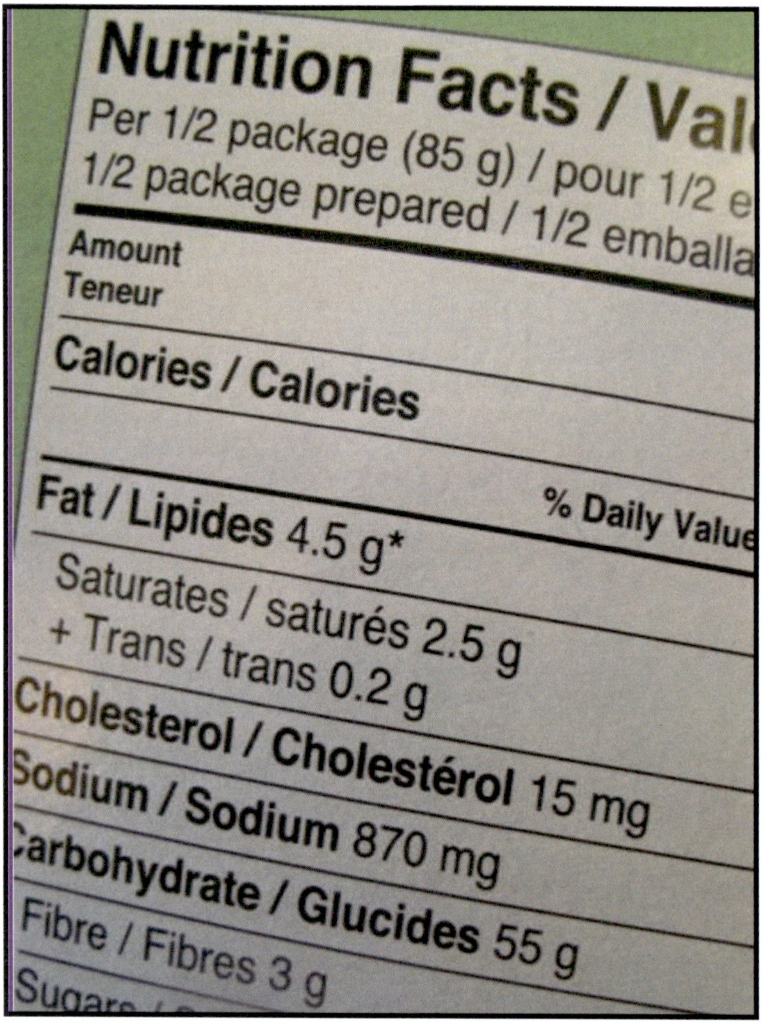
Nutrition Facts /
Per 1/2 package (85 g) / pour 1/2
1/2 package prepared / 1/2
Amount
Teneur
Calories / Calories
% Daily
Fat / Lipides 4.5 g*
Saturates / saturés 2.5 g
+ Trans / trans 0.2 g
Cholesterol / Cholestérol 15 mg
Sodium / Sodium 870 mg
Carbohydrate / Glucides 55 g
Fibre / Fibres 3 g

Gluten Foods

Gluten is a storage protein processed from wheat, barley and rye. It is commonly found in the majority of foods that have been commercially produced and processed. These may include: pastas, spaghetti, macaroni, pretzels, and bread or bread-based products, including pizza rolls, pizza crust, Stromboli. Baked goods, such as cookies, cakes and pies, are loaded with gluten. Prepared "so called" foods, such as frozen dinners, soups and casseroles, are also bloated with gluten. When making a choice to eat grains, such as wheat, barley and rye, these should only be consumed in their natural state. For example, wheatgrass is grown from the wheat berry itself and is considered non-gluten.

Common Additives to Release

These are the chemicals companies add to change the flavor, texture or substance of food, but add little nutritional or health value.

Look on the label for terms including: modified food starch, malt, hydrolyzed vegetable protein; vegetable gum and soy sauce. Read ALL product labels to determine which products are consistent with your choices, such as which are gluten-free and which are not.

Artificial Food Additives

Substances are added to food or food products to enhance flavor, taste and appearance. My rule of thumb: Avoid them all! This includes refined white sugar and other mini packs of sauces and add-ons that you may see at concession stands, coffee shops and restaurants. **Foods that contain artificial additives are not recommended for those who want to achieve and maintain optimal health and who desire maintaining a healthy weight.**

Alternative for Processed Sweeteners

Use raw honey, raw blue agave, or raw cane sugar. When you embrace these, you will then find other processed sweeteners to taste sticky and overpowering.

White Foods

The term "White Foods" applies to products, which are over processed. If you look at this list of common items in most kitchens, you can see where these products are more manufactured than harvested.

White Sugar: Your alternatives are raw honey or raw cane sugar (used in moderation).

White Flour: Your alternatives include coconut flour, almond flour, quinoa flour and millet flour. (Only found at Health Food Stores).

White Rice: Replace these with either quinoa seed, amaranth and teff grains.

White Bread: I recommend eliminating bread totally. For those who want a source while making this change, Ezekiel Bread is sprouted with an abundance of nutrients.

White Table Salt: Your best alternative is Pink Himalayan Salt. It has over 74 trace minerals and is an excellent source of sodium and other electrolytes, which are necessary minerals; and can be used in place of table salt. Additional choices for good salts: Celtic or sea salt.

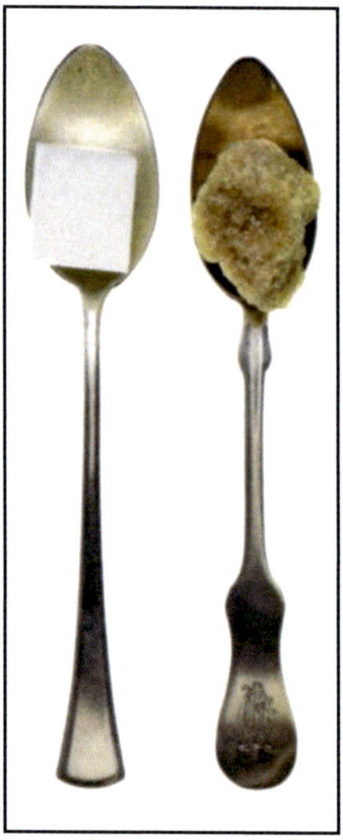

Fast Foods/Junk foods

There is no such thing as junk food - It's either 'food' or 'junk.' The human body only recognizes real foods and will try to find a way to get rid of the junk. What it can't get rid of, it stores in the body. Avoid eating fast foods and junk foods all together for Optimal Health!

Dairy

If you drink milk, here's a recommendation: purchase from a dairy farmer whom you trust and consume organic.

Milk Alternatives

Almond, hemp, and rice milks are good sources for Vitamin D and Calcium. Some contain 30% of each.

Other Healthy Beverages:

Enjoy herbal teas, fruit teas and fresh young coconut water (directly from coconut).

Cheese Alternatives

Cheese can be made from raw nuts, such as: cashews and can be a delicious alternative (A suggestion) look up recipes on YouTube.

Butter

Ghee vs. butter may be the best way to go as far as quality. Other alternatives include oils. *See oils & fats section on pages 33-34.*

Cereals

If you choose to eat cereals, you may want to consider organic. I advise to choose those, which are organic and have the least possible amounts of raw cane sugar. Totally avoid any cereals that contain regular or refined sugar. I also recommended avoiding the use of sweeteners in high amounts – measuring it any time you add something. When adding anything to foods, moderation is always the key. Aim to do what feels right for you and celebrate your victories! Forgive yourself and get back on track when you slip. Do better as you know better.

Vote With Your Dollars

Consider changing where you do business. It's a good idea to seek out natural health food stores, a naturopathic doctor, holistic dentist, alkaline water station and optional: natural hair salon, to assist you further on your wellness journey and new way of life. Also seek out raw food, vegan, vegetarian, Indian, middle-eastern and non-chain restaurants when possible.

Good Chain Restaurant Choices

If you must eat at a non-organic, chain restaurant:

Outback Steakhouse - Prepares everything fresh on site, unlike most other chain restaurants.

Other Alternatives for dining out (all have various locations)

La Marsa - Organic and Middle Eastern Cuisine

Chipotle Mexican Grill - Serves chicken and meat, which are free range and farmed within a 300 - mile radius in the state of Michigan! Serves organic fruit, veggies and black beans.

Reducing Food Waste

Have you ever thought about where your waste goes? In the big scheme of things, it all matters! Here's how the average U.S. citizen contributes to waste:

Food Waste: How often do you go out to eat, order too much and you end up leaving it on the table for waiter/waitress to throw away?

How often do you prepare/cook food, leave it out too long and throw it away?

Alternative

When ordering your meal in a restaurant, consider sharing your meal if you are dining out and maybe an appetizer for both of you. Another option: ask the waiter/waitress to bring a carryout box out with your meal and pack what you think you will not eat from the beginning.

Usually a meal portion while dining out is double the actual serving size of a recommended portion. The most effective answer is to just cut it in half. This has two wins for you: it helps you maintain portion control and stretches your food dollar by creating two meals from one.

When preparing and cooking at home, work, going to parties/events or a friend's home, have reusable storage containers ready to pack food up you will not eat right away and store them out of sight in the refrigerator.

Boosting Your Metabolism Naturally

Organic Apple Cider Vinegar

I truly believe organic apple cider vinegar is a life saver and life enhancer! For many years people have been including organic apple cider vinegar in their diet and it can have infinite benefits on your health! In order to reap the many benefits, be sure to only buy organic in a glass bottle with the cloudy film at the bottom of liquid. Properties organic apple cider vinegar includes: vitamins, minerals, antioxidants, fiber, enzymes and organic acids.

I often drink a teaspoon in a glass of water on an empty stomach (best done in morning). This can enhance energy level and balance body weight. I also sprinkle on top of my salads and use to soak non-organic fruit and vegetables with added water.

My experience with adding a teaspoon of Bragg's organic apple cider vinegar has been: increased energy, more alertness, weight management and increased metabolism! There are also many other benefits to drinking Bragg's apple cider vinegar!

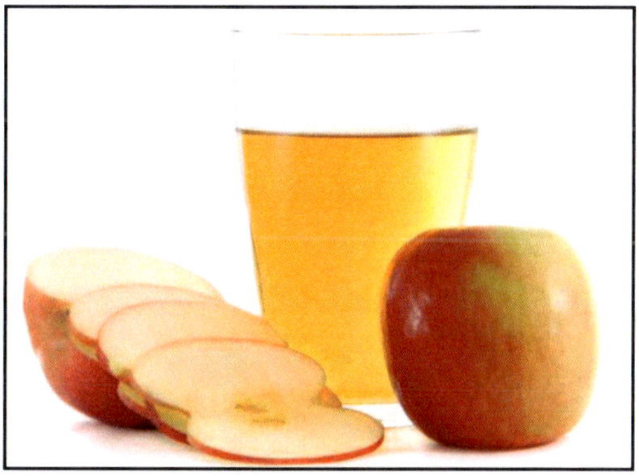

For more information on the many more benefits of organic apple cider vinegar visit: **www.bragg.com**

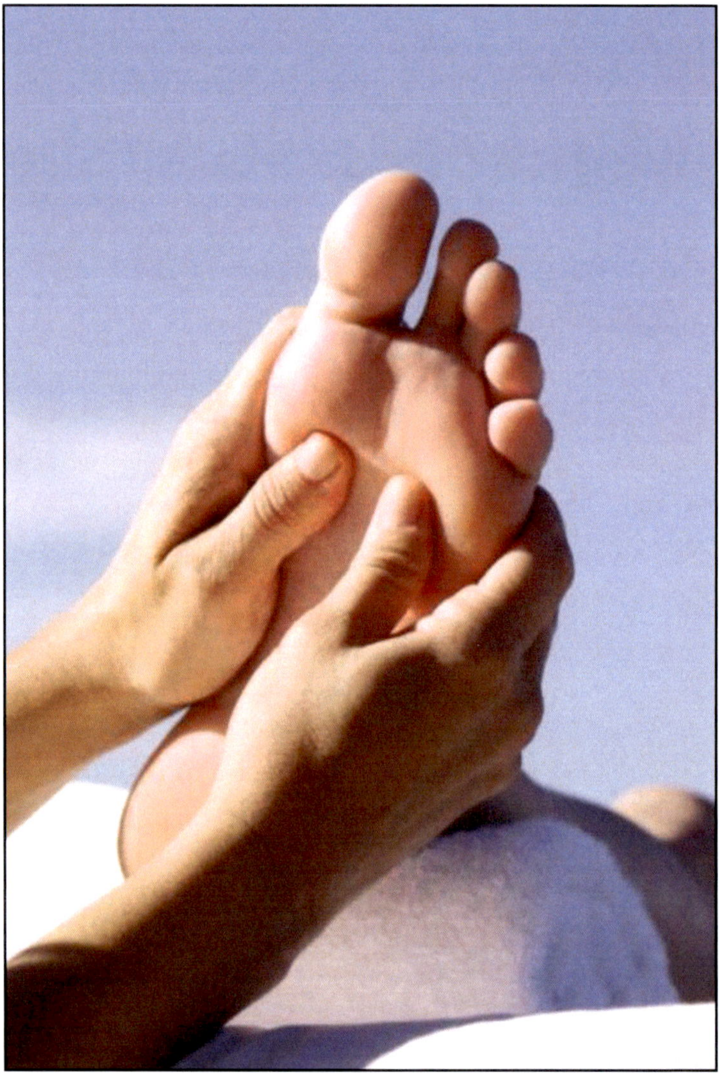

Digestion and Colon Health

Digestion

To achieve Optimal Health and digestion, I recommend that you eat as many foods as possible, in their raw and natural state. Central to this are leafy greens, fruit, vegetables, sprouted beans, lentils, grains, raw nuts and seeds. In addition, consistently consuming prunes, raisins and apples may help you to stay regular.

Although the process of digestion starts in the mouth, with our salvia, this alone is not enough to process large amounts of cooked foods or large molecules of meat. As mentioned above, we need help from digestive enzymes! If you do not eat a lot of raw foods, it's essential to supplement your diet with digestive enzymes. My personal preference is **Enzymedica's Digest Gold**. They should be taken with each meal.

Get Moving!

The digestive process is actually three processes: Ingestion, Digestion, and Egestion or Elimination. Many people are uncomfortable talking about the last one. It's so important to be active in order to be regular. Choose something that interests you that you can stick to by yourself. This can include walking, jogging, bike riding or other forms of exercise! Find a partner to exercise, dance or go walking or jogging together.

Regular Therapeutic Massage

Hands on and Migun Bed Massages have many benefits to them. These help with pain reduction, great lymphatic movement, circulation and other benefits to the body. They may help your total digestive process.

Here is an important self-nurturing technique I have found to be highly valuable: Massage the inside of your hands and bottom of feet every day, to assist with elimination. These key areas are connected to the organs in your body, including your intestines! In addition, take the time to massage around your abdomen to help more with elimination.

For more information about Migun bed massage, visit this website: www.migunworld.com

Fiber and Colon Health

If you require assistance with cleaning out your colon or to remain regular; I have found great success with taking Now Brand Organic psyllium whole husks mixed in water.

Enemas

Enemas are a very helpful therapy when done correctly. My experience has shown me that moderate use of enemas will help with keeping the colon clean and when constipation occurs.

I have found great success with the following method:

- Purchase an enema 2-4 bottle kit, pour out contents then rinse.
- Wipe off nozzle with dry cloth and apply Shea butter or olive oil.
- Pour in alkaline or purified water and add a small amount of powdered Spirulina , small amount of liquid wheat grass or parsley juice

By performing this, the enema will loosen up the waste material to eliminate on the walls of the intestinal tract. Regular use can actually tone up and nourish intestine walls.

Elimination

The human body was designed to eliminate waste after each meal 2-3 times per day is absolutely normal for Optimal Health!

As I mentioned in the introduction, I had my gall bladder removed when I was young. If you are like me and do not have a gall bladder, you may experience a challenge with digestion as I do from time to time. I have found when I eat more raw leafy dark greens, such as: Kale, Chard, and Turnip Greens ("Yes you can eat these Raw or put them in your smoothie or juice them"), my experience is that my overall digestion is easier, as well as my bowel movements. For me, it is so essential to eat more raw foods ,if you do not have a gall bladder! If your body does not allow you to eat them raw, they can also be lightly steamed.

I have found great success when I commit to a 3-10 day raw fruit, vegetable and juice fast from time to time. As with any diet, always check with your Medical or Natural Doctor before going on any diet.

While I have given you my best recommendations, some of you will still have fast food as a part of your diet. If you are someone who still chooses to eat junk foods, I highly recommend that you balance this out by, taking digestive enzymes and getting a colonic every once in a while. Look up your local holistic clinic and ask them. I have found this will aid the total digestive process if you still make junk or processed food choices.

Poop

Pay attention to this important body system to monitor.

Ideally, healthy poop should be smooth and 8-12 inches long. Anything else may indicate a diet change need, releasing of drugs, alcohol, cigarettes, fast foods etc. Digestive enzymes and raw leafy greens also help to have healthy poop.

The next page is a reference guide which will help tell you more about what's going on inside of you.

How Do You Doo Chart

What Should an Ideal Bowel Movement Look and Smell Like?

An ideal bowel movement (IBM) is medium brown and should look like type 4. A IBM should happen 3 times a day and be approximately 4 to 8 inches long. IBM should be in one piece, like the shape and size of a banana and tapered at the end. IBM should leave the body easily with no straining or discomfort. There should be little to no gas or odor. IBM should not take more than a minute to completely evacuate.

The seven common types of stools per the Bristol Stool Chart are:

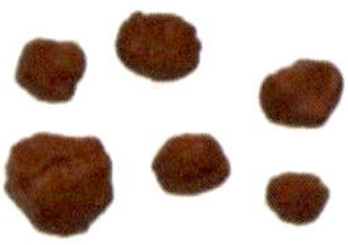

Type 1: separate hard lumps, like nuts (hard to pass). Constipation- even if you're defecating frequently. Not enough water. Possible causes are eating too much dry food, including protein, and not enough vegetables and raw foods, laxative abuse, worries, or irritable bowel syndrome.

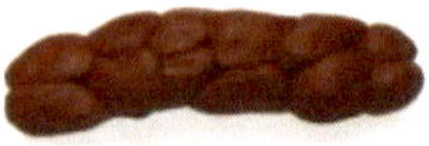

Type 2: sausage-shaped but lumpy. This type is also constipation. See type 1 for same causes.

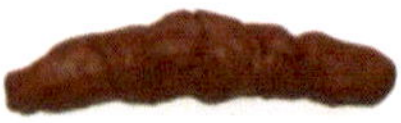

Type 3: like a sausage but with cracks on its surface = optimal

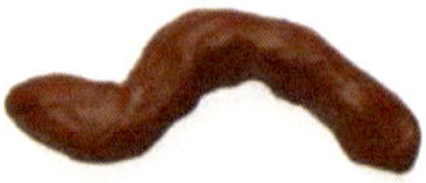

Type 4: like a sausage or snake, smooth and soft = Ideal way to pass. This is our goal to achieve, when having a BM.

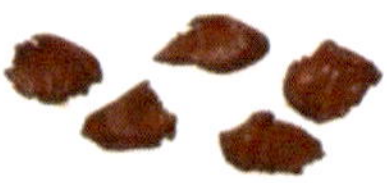

Type 5: soft blobs with clear-cut edges, easily passed through digestive system. Soft diarrhea- may indicated a possible risk for bowel disease. You also may be toxic and need a intestinal cleansing.

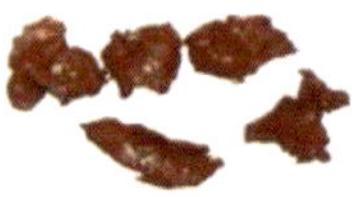

Type 6: fluffy pieces with ragged edges, a mushy stool/diarrhea- indicated you may be toxic and need a intestinal cleansing.

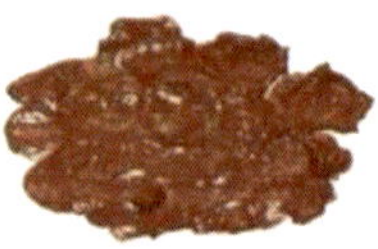

Type 7: loose, watery, no solid pieces, and sometimes can see undigested foods Diarrhea- possible causes are food, poisoning lactose intolerance, antibiotics, antacids, dietary changes, travel, anxiety, stress, inflammatory bowel disease, or irritable bowel syndrome.

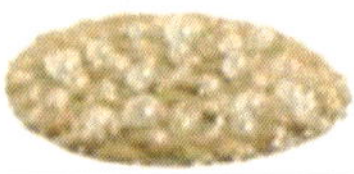

Type 8: stool has a mucous-like consistency, with bubbles and foul odor. This may indicate unsafe amounts of alcohol and/or recreational drugs.

The Bristol Stool Chart was first published in the Scandinavian Journal of Gastroenterology in 1997. This version is a compilation and hand illustrated by the Kimbrell Family with clay. LivingAnointed.com

Female Health

Remedies for Maintaining Good Vaginal Health

**Proceed using your inner guidance*

My experience has been, when I wear cotton underwear I feel better. Your underwear and clothing should allow your body to breathe. Also, I do not use any powders or fragrances in the private area; because they are not necessary and they may cause irritation. Be as natural as you can and you will reap the benefits!

Douching for freshness, keeping female organs toned, nourished and helps with balancing Yeast/Candida or Bacteria infections. I have been successful using the following as different options:

- Purchase a douche 2-4 bottle kit, pour out contents and rinse thoroughly
- Pour in alkaline or purified water and add a small amount of powdered Spirulina or a *small amount of liquid wheat grass or parsley juice
- Coconut water is also an option with nothing added

Vaginal Suppositories Recipe

- Have small glass measuring cup handy
- Melt Spectrum unrefined coconut oil with a few drops of rosemary essential oil
- Stir, mix well and let cool
- Pour into suppositories and freeze for 1 hour
- Take out as needed and insert into vagina

- Use only at bedtime, Wear a panty liner to protect both your underwear and bed linens.

Other fungal infections include:

Jock itch and athlete's foot

My personal experience for preventing/releasing Candida or yeast infection:

If you want to maintain good vaginal flora balance, steer clear of added sweeteners such as: agaves, honey, refined and cane sugars, carbonated beverages, processed foods, junk foods, fast foods, sweets other than natural fruit, foods with additives/preservatives etc. Also, never use perfumes, body powder, deodorant sprays or anything else near your vaginal area. It's recommended that you also wear only cotton underwear; and to go a step further, organic cotton is always better! Find on-line. This is also good to balance good flora in your gut and vagina.

Raw Garlic: A Strong and Natural Antibiotic

My experience taught me the healing power of raw garlic. It helped to get rid of an aggressive yeast infection and here's how. I bought a pack of raw garlic, peeled one clove per day and ate it throughout the day for 2 weeks. At the end of that time, the symptoms went away and the yeast infection was totally gone! As an added by-product, I found my sense of taste had cleared up!

I find it to be the best practice to mince up the clove into small pieces. Start out with a tiny piece so that your body can get used to it. I also took small pieces and wrapped them inside of my leafy greens or raw parsley and chewed them. I did this with every meal. I recommend to thoroughly chewing the raw garlic before you eat

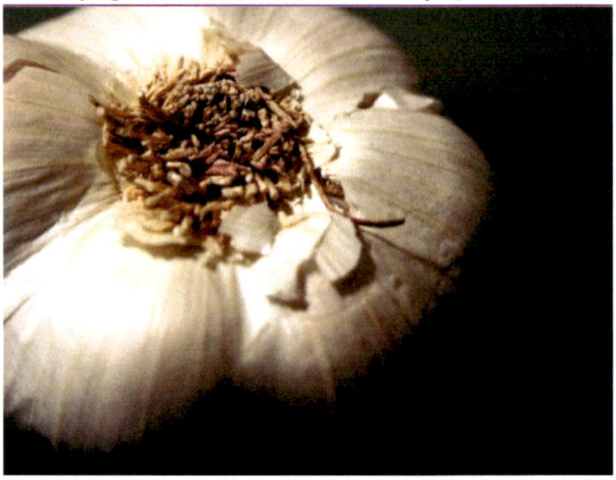

your meal with the leafy greens or parsley. Then it's optional to also add pieces to your actual meal.

There is a bi-product which you should know about. Your underarms may have a slight or strong odor for a time, depending on what type of deodorant you use, because you will be detoxing your body by this process. You may also have a pronounced breath odor. I have found it may be helpful to chew raw parsley immediately afterwards or keep a therapeutic grade peppermint spray on you to freshen up your breath.

Personally for me, I did not care if I smelled like garlic or not. I just wanted the infection gone! I can report outstanding results.

Another option as a strong remedy is to use **Inner Defense.** This is a capsule that **Young Living** distributes. Along with this protocol, would be to also get a good Probiotic, such as **Live 5** from **Young Living** as well and can be taken at night.

Sex and Candida/Yeast Infection

One of the biggest myths in medicine is that men do not get yeast or Candida infections. This is not true! In fact, it is men who can pass it on to women through sexual intercourse! If you are in a sexual relationship, both partners should follow the protocol!

Annual Woman's Medical Exam

A tip for ladies when getting your annual pap smear - always take your own lubricant. Aloe Vera Gel without preservatives is an excellent choice! I also have found it to be a good idea to douche afterwards. If you already have a condition, the ingredients in the commercial grade lubricant your OB-GYN uses may irritate it even more! Aloe Vera gel can also be used in place of commercial lubricants with synthetics for vaginal dryness during intercourse.

Natural Contraceptive Considerations

I stopped taking birth control pills around age 28. One day I woke up and intuitively knew they were not good for my body and ceased using them. To me the side effects just weren't worth it.

If you set the intention to remain without child, this is what your experience can be. If you worry about becoming pregnant, you may attract it into your experience. Being in tune with your body, mind & spirit can help you tune in to the rhythm of your body and to know when it is safe to engage in sex. The next option would be to know when your ovulation period is, and according to this, choose when it's safe for you to have sex. You can also obtain a calendar/chart on-line or from your OB-GYN, of how the ovulation process works.

Another option might be to use neem oil, which I have used. It is 100% natural and when inserted into the vagina and or rubbed on the tip of penis prior to intercourse; it may protect from pregnancy. This form of birth control is used in India. You may want to do your own research. The final alternative would be to use condoms of your choice.

Menstrual Cycle

Years ago I used to experience cramps when it was that time of the month. PMS is a hormone related condition and the goal is to give the body what it needs, so this does not occur. Then I went on an 80% raw food diet and started eating lots of raw, organic greens, fruit and veggies and more particularly, I ate lots of berries! Black berries, blueberries & strawberries. I also drank fresh coconut water and the cramps vanished! You especially want to eliminate the consumption of artificial sweeteners and soda pop.

There was no pre-cramping or anything before it would come on, it just showed up! This told me something, that foods we eat, do affect our health! Cramping during your menstrual cycle is not normal, especially if they are severe! Remember that pain is one way our bodies let us know something is wrong or the body being out of Balance!

During your menstrual cycle, your body is releasing and cleansing itself. Along with this process, your body looses minerals. If you are already depleted, you really need to replenish and be consistent with taking your multi-vitamins and minerals; especially calcium!

In addition, I have found peppermint and lavender essential oils to be very helpful for cramps! When needed, I just apply a drop or 2 on my abdomen area. Allowing time to care for you during this time is essential. It also helped me to drink herbal teas to soothe myself. Some good ones are nettles, peppermint and red clover.

Embracing you at any age

Your body was designed to balance itself out, at all ages. As you continue to nurture yourself and follow info. in this book, you can continue to enjoy your life! As an added benefit to what's in this book; I keep my hormones balanced by using essential oils and I can feel that I have enough estrogen & progesterone. I pay attention to how I feel at all times! **there is also a creme called progesterone that is worth checking out online.**

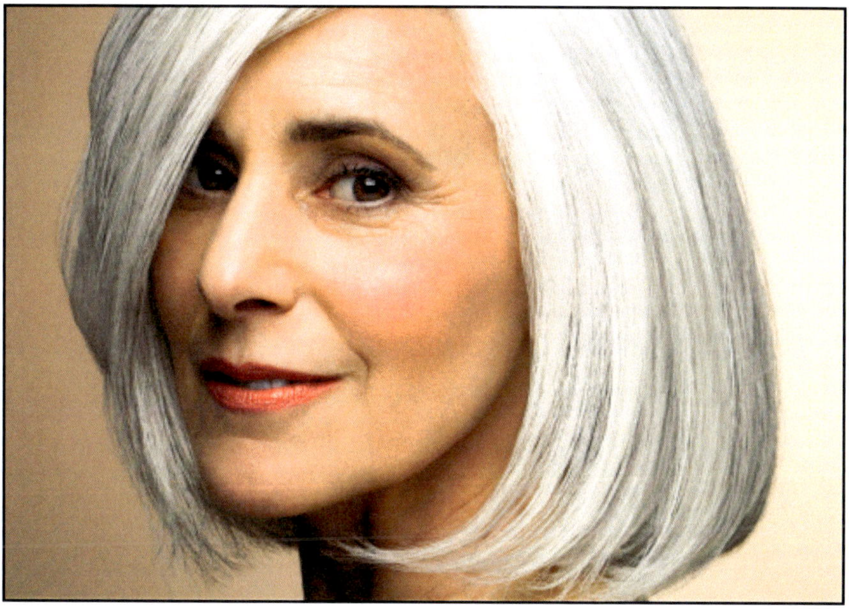

Thyroid Health

The Thyroid is the Energy gland of the human body and produces T3 and T4 Thyroid hormones that control the body's metabolism. It also controls other vital functions such as digestion, circulation, immune function, hormone balance and emotions.

Source: Essential Oils pocket reference 5th Edition

I had a former office position, which the office was fairly small. My work area was next to a large printer, which was always in use. Because of inhaling the toner from the printer, it threw my thyroid out of balance! Within 2 months, I started experiencing symptoms of the following: missed periods, digestion and constipation issues and minor challenges when it came to swallowing. In order to have bowel movements, at times I had to do colon cleanses 1-2 times per day and dong enemas. This went on for 2 months. Then my friend Joy started teaching me about essential oils and came to my rescue! Shortly after, I ordered my essential oils kit. When I received my essential oil kit in the mail, one of the blended oils is called Valor. Without reading any information about this oil, I intuitively knew to apply it to my thyroid area, so I did. Within 2 weeks of using Valor the symptoms went away and my thyroid was back into balance! Thank God for essential oils!

Health Indicators

Eye Health

Our eyes tell us a lot about our health. If your eyes are clear (cornea), it's a good sign of having a clean diet and healthy body. It they are cloudy, beige, or has lines etc. it could be an indication to change your diet or to release the consumption or use of toxic chemicals, smoking and or alcohol consumption. It may also be a good idea to start a detox regimen.

Nails

Our nails are another way the body lets us know about our health.

Nails should be clear with white half-moon at bottom near the cuticle. They should also be strong, free of streaks, white spots and dents. When I experienced the above, I started taking **New Chapter** bone strength & multi-vitamin for women (they have multi for men also), **Now** vitamin D3 and putting **ConcenTrace Minerals** in my water daily. & or rubbing **Derma MAG** on bottom of my feet at night.

I am also sure to eat a healthy diet and use natural body care and household products. Starting with internal health helps to maintain the health of areas like finger and toe nails.

Best Practices

Best Refrigerator for preserving foods (may preserve food longer) Kitchen Aid French Door Refrigerator

Suggested items to purchase

Glass Storing Bowls with lids
Glass Cutting Board
(Washes clean without bacteria)
Mason Jars (store smoothies, juices etc
Coffee Grinder
(Used to grind seeds into powders)
Set of sharp knives
Food Processor (optional)
Timer
Blender, Black and Decker
(With glass) or
NutriBullet www.nutribullet.com
at Lexan Manual Juicer
(Used for juicing wheatgrass, parsley etc.) and other juicing machines.
Order here: www.wheatgrasshome.com

Spices

Spices are an important part of every meal. They add great flavor and can enhance any meal. Furthermore, they have medicinal properties. If you use them often, you can buy them in bulk whenever possible at health food stores.

Of course, they can be purchased at the grocery store in jars. However, you explore more at T.J. Maxx, Marshall's and Burlington Coat Factory, along with Superfoods!

Other Edibles

Flowers and Wild Herbs - Check at your local Farmer's Market. Become a student - buy books and learn about them!

Household Cleaners & more

The following can be used in place of commercial household products which contain toxic chemicals. These gifts made with ingredients from nature can add cleaning power to your everyday chores!

- **Young Living** Thieves Cleaning Kit
- **Seventh Generation** Dish Soap, laundry detergent & cleaning products
- Borax and Baking Soda mixed (for cleaning and laundry)
- MMS **(Miracle Mineral Solution)** kills germs and pathogens and can be used on White Laundry, Dishes, clean counter tops, floors, toilet etc. *(some people ingest it to expel parasites, be sure to do your own research).*

Dr. Jim Bumble discovered it.

Order here: www.mmsdrops.com/great-home-uses-for-mms

Cooking and Cookware Alternative

I recommend as a first choice to use a slow cooker whenever possible for cooking anything, instead of baking or frying my second choice is to use glass or ceramic with glass or ceramic lids. A third option is stainless steel. Avoid non-stick chemical coated cookware, which release these compounds into the foods while cooking.

Use toaster oven instead of conventional oven to take the chill off foods (heating). Remember the goal is to reduce over-heating your foods as much as possible; to preserve vital enzymes and nutrients!

Education is Powerful!

Watch Movies and Documentaries that tell you the stories behind the foods you eat. Check with your local library or on Netflix and check out these titles: Supersize Me, Food Inc., The Corporation and Tapped.

Highly Recommended Books:

- Natural Cures they don't want You to know about, by: Kevin Treduau
- Recipes for Longer Life by: Ann Wigmore
- Essential Oils Pocket Reference, 5th Edition
- Fountain of Youth by: Peter Kelder
- You can Heal your Life by: Louise L. Hay
- Getting into the Vortex Meditations, by: Abraham Hicks

Websites:

Take the time to research what's important to you. If desired, find out below how much nutrition is in the foods you eat. Also, there is a free on-line diet and weight reduction journal included.

www.nutritiondata.self.com

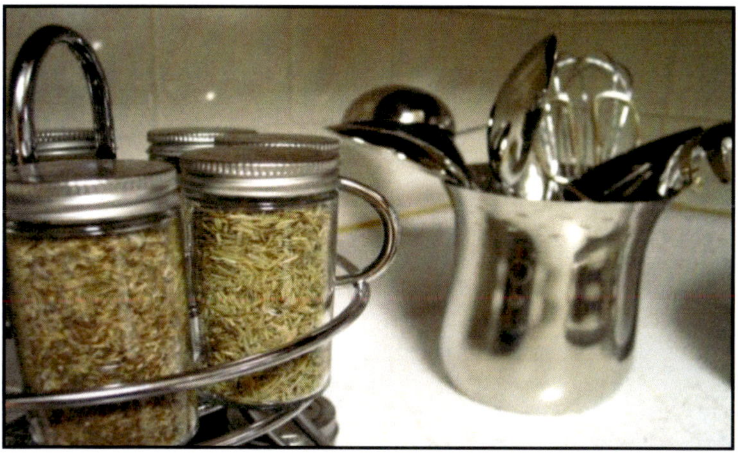

Body Care Choices

How many millions of dollars are spent each year by people who think that the well-advertised hygiene products are their best choices? As a part of your shift, take the time to invest in your well-being and follow these simple recipes for a healthy alternative. Following recommendations of this lifestyle guide will be of great assistance.

Natural Deodorant

You can purchase natural and effective deodorant which contains sodium bicarbonate.

You may want to sew in a panel of cotton, in your shirts, to absorb excess sweat if you wear natural deodorant. Works well if your shirt is made from cotton or thick blend of fabric.

Body Moisturizer Recipe

- **Organic unrefined coconut oil**
- **Almond oil (optional)**
- **Unrefined shea butter**
- **Few drops of your favorite essential oil**

You can get additional ideas if you go to YouTube and search for natural hair and body moisturizers.

Oral Care

Toothpaste

I prefer Nature's Gate Peppermint toothpaste. While it is generally available at health food stores, look for the best prices at places such as Kroger, in the organic section of store.

Mouthwash

Why pay inflated prices when you can simply and affordably make your own. You will need: Young Living Clove essential oil, alkaline water and a small glass bottle(s) with tops to them. This essential oil is about $14 (plus shipping) and will last for months

Naturally Whiten Teeth

Although white strips may be poplar, they may not be the healthiest. My experience with them: the can strip enamel from your teeth and make them sensitive. Instead, I use **Nature's Gate** toothpaste and an organic banana from time to time. Be sure to wash banana peel thoroughly, then use inside of peel and scrub teeth with. I usually do it for 2-3min. You will see a noticeable result immediately!

Also, when getting your teeth cleaned, you can take your own (All Natural mouthwash) or request that your dental hygienist order All Natural products for your visit. Another option is to find a Wholistic Dentist in your area.

Oil Pulling

Oil pulling is an ancient remedy practiced by many, who want to improve the health of their gums and teeth. The process is thought to pull toxins from the body. I have seen videos of people's gums when receding and were starting to be restored as early as 2 weeks! Other benefits may be: tighten teeth, reduce or eliminate gum and teeth sensitivity & so much more!

How I use it & what I use

- Purchase unrefined coconut oil or unrefined sesame oil
- Measure a tablespoon or close to it and put inside mouth
- Swish around & hold for 10 - 20 seconds, then spit out.

Testimonial:

Katina helped me save my teeth by recommending oil pulling & supplements. My desire to smoke cigarettes also decreased! I went from smoking a pack a day to just 6 per day now!! ~Hugh McGuire

Skincare and Hair Care

Use products that are as natural as possible. Here are a few trusted brands I use: **Nature's Gate** from **Kroger** – reasonably priced – (in organic section), **Everyone** by: **EO** – reasonably priced – from **Whole Foods Market, Origins** and **Aveda** (Nationwide locations)

Natural Breath Fresheners

Young Living Peppermint Essential Oil, just one drop will do. Keep in mind I recommend this brand simply because it is pure. Be Aware, other brands may not be pure or safe to be taken by mouth. Another option is to use **fresh cloves** and you would only need to break off a small piece. *Just be aware, it may be a bit strong or hot until you get used to the flavor.*

Chewing Gum Option

The best option is, to get chewing form a health food store or the brand **Spry.** This brand uses Xylitol as a sweetener; which is naturally found in low concentrations in the fibers of fruit and vegetables.

Hair Care

Ever consider going Natural? There are many benefits to this including the absence of toxic chemicals. Did you know everything you put on your scalp is absorbed into your brain and the whole body? When toxic chemicals are used, they cause disruption to the cells in the body; which can lead to generative dis-ease.

Henna Hair Dye

This is all natural from the Henna plant, and many Indian women use it for hair dye as well as body tattoos/ body art. It is a great way to naturally color your hair and use as a rinse! I absolutely love henna!

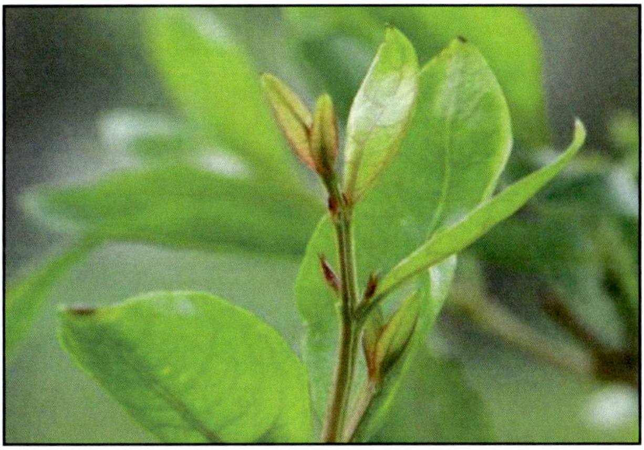

Find more information on YouTube.

Natural Makeup

Natural is the way to go! You can choose from an array of shades in pressed powders, eye shadow, blush, eyeliners, lip sticks and lip glosses! Ingredients should be mostly plant based. Where to buy: **Aveda, Origins** and **Bare Minerals** in numerous locations.

Also, grocery stores and just about every department store now carries natural makeup. Some of the price points are about the same as other makeup brands and are healthier, in my opinion.

Facial Care

Two great places to shop for facial and body care for all skin types are **Aveda and Origins** in malls across the U.S. Here are a few options. My first choice for caring for my face (oily skin), is the line called 'Zero Oil' made by Origins. Another choice is Aloe Vera shampoo (I use on my face) by Nature's Gate.

Eyebrows

If you arch your eyebrows, here's a tip to get them to lie them down and be smooth. Apply a small amount of **Nature's Gate** tea tree shampoo. If you are considering coloring your eyebrows, natural Henna color from the Henna plant may be a great choice!

Dry Skin Brushing

This is also another ancient remedy that has been used for centuries! It can have profound benefits on your overall health! It may also help to prevent conditions. When dry skin-brushing is done on a regular basis, along with consuming Alkaline Water, eating a diet as clean & healthy as possible, sunshine, proper rest/sleep, and exercise.

A way to do this is buy and start using an All Natural dry skin brush from your local health store. As you include this awesome remedy in your daily regimen, notice the positive effects it has on your health; including better skin appearance.

Only dry skin brush where skin is healthy, strong and free of rashes, bruises, sores etc. Some bodily areas are more sensitive than others, so use less pressure in these areas.

Here's how: I dry skin brush in the morning before showering (while skin is dry and pores are still closed), take your dry-skin brush and stroke from your hands and up your arms and also starting near your ankles and up your legs toward the heart, stroking on each side of arms and legs, even under the arms. I also dry skin brush in the evening before bedtime.

Benefits:

- Dry skin brushing can help your body get rid of dead skin cells and make room for new skin cell growth and maintain its healthy glow, smoother skin and youthful appearance!

- Helps skin and pores to breathe better
- It is the largest organ of the body & helps with whole-body function
- Increases circulation and enhances immune system
- Improves drainage of lymph in the skin and remove toxins from shin

- Helps to minimize cellulite (which are toxins stored in tissue).
- Helps to distribute body weight and I noticed more muscle tone
- Stimulates hormone and oil glands. Keep in mind dry skin brushing is helping your lymph system and whole-body to move & exercise itself and helping everything to flow better
- Since all of the body is connected, dry skin brushing helps the whole-body to Function better and help to boost energy levels
- There are also many more benefits. I know for sure, dry skin brushing has truly enhanced my health.
- Pregnant & nursing women have also been known to benefit from dry skin brush. However, lighter strokes may be necessary. ***Do your own research and listen to your body.***
- May be safe for children also. My 6 year young nephew loves it.
- Most health food stores carry natural dry skin brushes. They come mostly wooden with a long handle and natural Brussels and some of the bases are detachable; which makes it even more convenient.

Care for Dry Skin Brushes

- Make sure that you clean them at least once per month. I usually immerse into warm water with Nature's Gate tea tree shampoo and scrub with fingers.
- When done scrubbing, rinse well, shake off excess water and allow to air dry
- Never share your dry skin brush with anyone. Everyone should have their own.
- Keep in dry place and away from moisture.

Rough and Dry Skin

A good moisturizer is necessary to have smooth and healthy skin. The skin is the largest organ in the body. It is Essential to use only products made from nature! I have great success with making and using my own body butter.

I use it all over the body, with the exception of my face; because I have oily skin. If you do not want to make your own, you can purchase body butters

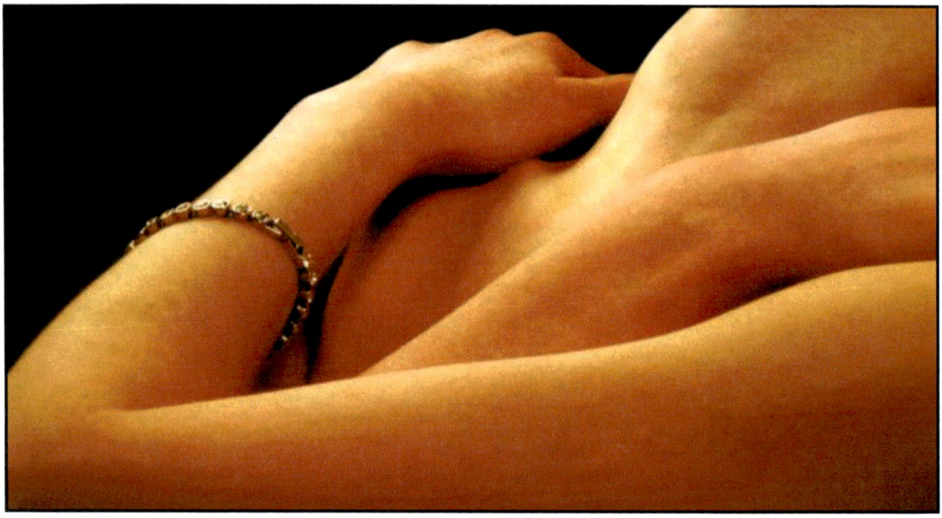

and lotions from a health food store, **Whole Foods Market, Plum Market, Better Health, Aveda** or **Origins.**

Scaly Feet/Dead Skin

You will need:

- Hand towel
- Dish washing pan
- Himalayan Salt or Sea Salt
- Pumice or Long Rectangle nail file (from beauty supply store)
- Water enough to completely cover both feet (Alkaline is best)

Prepare warm water, then add small amount of Pink Himalayan Salt or Sea Salt and soak 15-30min. This will cause dead skins to come off the bottom of the feet. Rub and massage feet to remove dead skin. Repeat as often as necessary.

Happy Feet Maintenance

Be sure to take care of your feet, they carry you everywhere you want to go! Also your organs inside your body are connected to your feet! Read more about **Reflexology** on-line.

To maintain smooth and happy feet, it's recommended to always wear comfortable shoes, with thick soles. High heeled shoes should only be worn on occasion. I have found that high heeled wedged shoes or sandals give more support than other high heeled shoes. Fashion should never replace comfort! Make it a point to invest in comfortable shoes; they can take you a long way with your health! When bottom of feet start to get scaly, file them with the nail file mentioned above.

Wear All Natural or Organic Cotton Clothes

Cotton is my favorite fabric to wear, because it actually comes from a plant! I love how it feels on my skin and I have more clothing in this fabric, than any other fabric.

For my underwear, this is the only way to go! Also, it allows your body to breathe! Also keep in mind that many clothing types contain dye, which you may be able to smell or feel; if they were not properly treated beforehand put on the market.

For instance black and dark blue jeans may sometime run or smear on a light colored shirt. This may be especially true when shopping a discount department store, where clothing is sold because of minor defects.

For this reason, I do not wear darker colored jeans, unless they are somewhat faded.

Shop at **Whole Foods Market** and online.

Baby Care

***Proceed using your inner guidance**

Feeding

According to Medical Director Tarah Colaizy, breast feeding is the optimal way to feed your baby and there are a lot of health benefits associated with breast feeding with both moms and babies. Human breast milk is especially beneficial to pre-mature babies! The 2nd best choice is donor's breast milk. Third choice is Goat's milk. The consistency of (unpasteurized) Goats Milk is similar to skim milk and has a light flavor. The most amounts of nutrients, enzymes and protein are bio available, when milk is raw (unpasteurized). However, when heated (pasteurized) the above are still much better choices.

Other Alternatives

These include: **Meyenberg Whole Powdered Goats Milk.** Check at your local health food store, **Whole Foods Market** or order online.
It has been my experience that when soothing baby after feeding, to rub baby's back instead of patting. Babies are gentle and should be handled with care at all times including when (burping) or soothing after feeding.

Mothers Breast Milk Bank

The University of Iowa Alumni started a Mother's Milk Bank 11 years ago and is the 5th on record to start one! There are 15 donation depots throughout the state of Iowa, to help make sure that newborns will grow to become healthy children! You can research this on YouTube.

If you are a healthy newborn baby mother who produces a high volume of milk, you may want to consider becoming a donor!

Skincare

Generally All Natural oils and butters are safe for babies such as: almond oil, grape seed oil, coconut oil, olive oil and shea butter.

Essential oils

Certain essential oils are said to be safe for babies, such as: lavender and gentle baby. Many people I know have told me it's ok to let babies smell them between ages 0-6mo. Beyond this age, others have put just a drop or 2 on bottom of babies feet. Be sure to do your own research on this!

You can google and watch YouTube videos to find out what others have done. I also highly recommend ordering the book: **Gentle Baby** on Amazon.

Note: If you plan to go outdoors in the Spring/Summer time or if you live/travel in a warm climate, do not use the oils, because bees like them, too!

Baby Bottom Recipe

These might be helpful with relieving diaper rash:

- Spectrum, organic unrefined coconut oil (alone) or mix with
- Unrefined shea butter
- Few drops of lavender essential oil

If mixing these ingredients, find out *how* on YouTube! Also, to get more recipes and recipe ideas for making your own *natural moisturizers*.

Animal Care

Quality Products

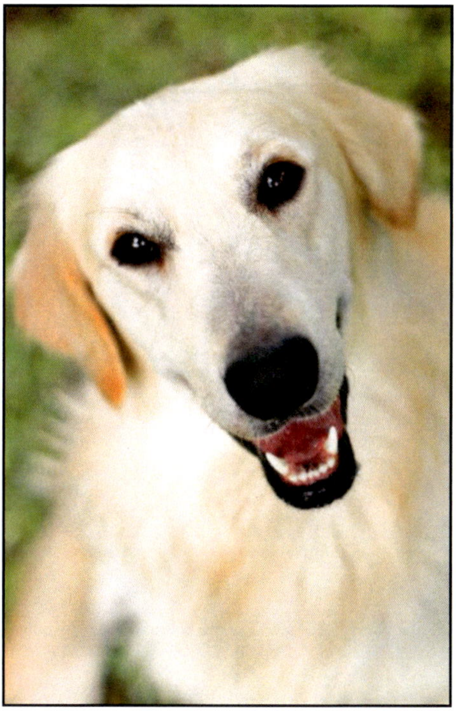

Consider your pet when improving your own lifestyle. Consider giving your dog or cat premium dog or cat food. This would include both a mixture of dry and moist dog or cat foods, with all natural ingredients. Dry foods alone; do not provide them with all the nutrients their bodies require. The same goes if you have other animals such as: birds, guinea pig or conditioned outdoor animals.

Give them the best foods for whatever species they are and, only use natural products around them (for cleaning etc.) The air they breathe is important also. Get familiar with reading ingredient labels and choose brands that have the most (real food) ingredients as possible! Or make homemade food for them and not your leftovers! Research and find out what works for them! Also, dogs and cats like to be in nature, no matter what the season is. It's a good idea, to allow your dog or cat time outdoors in nature and to run freely.

Proper Pet Care

If you have a dog, ideally there is an area for it to run freely that is safe for it as well as other people who may be in the area. Perhaps, if it is trained well and harmless, you can take your pet to a nearby park for recreation. Some Young Living essential oils are safe for pets, just like they are humans. They are creatures from nature as well and when The Creator intended our medicine to come from nature, the same is true for them!

Animals are more intuitive that most humans and they know when to go outside and eat grass (their natural medicine) when their bodies need it! Also, please only use natural cleaning and other products around your pets and the areas they live in.

A Healthier Home

Thinking of having your own house built?

This has many advantages to it! You get to design it according to your taste and select the materials you like!

There are also other advantages, from an environmental standpoint. You can choose what type of flooring you want; Example: Hardwood floors or untreated carpeting. You can decide on either a high ceiling with Solar Panels. Maybe you can purchase acres of land with lots of trees etc. Wherever you go consider having your very own garden! This can be an advantage because the more land you have around you, the more seeds you can plant for your garden! You can also get your neighbors involved and start a community garden!

Solar Panels

I love the idea of saving money on electric bills and being off the grid. Also Imagining the Magnificent rays of the Sunlight! Did you know the Sun is our main Energy Source on planet earth? Power plants are only vehicles, which deliver the energy you use. How about getting it directly from the Source? Solar panels allow the Solar Rays to come into your home or office; therefore you would not need as much energy from your electric company! Depending on where you live, and how much you see the sun, year around.

Cellular phones, iPods and other electronic items, can also be charged using a Solar Charger. Visit Amazon and type in Solar Chargers for more information.

Harmonize Your Home

Are you aware, many consumer electronics used daily give off radiation and are not good for your health? This can come from cell phones, cordless phones, microwaves, video game consoles, refrigerators and more! All these have different levels of radiation.

How to remedy this: Daily prayer, meditation, deep breathing, positive music therapy, eating a balanced diet, deep breathing, sunshine, alkaline water and essential oils and Spirulina can all help to raise your immune system! When your immune system is strong, it protects you from elements that may be harmful.

Microwaves give off much radiation. I have not used a microwave in over 10 years! When you start to heat your food using a conventional or toaster oven, it will taste so much better and more nutrients will be preserved!

Air Freshener

All Natural therapeutic grade essential oils and diffuser are great choices for keeping home environment clean, fresh and free of toxins.

Let me recommend investing in the Premium Starter Kit. In the kit, you can get 10 scented therapeutic grade essential oils and home diffuser. This will allow you an array of fragrant therapeutic grade essential oils and diffuser for your home or office. Also having the diffuser and essential oils, can allow you to experience the natural aroma of the oils throughout your home and can be a mood enhancer! One of the oils includes Thieves, which is a blended oil which kills mold inside the home.

Must Have Appliances: Irons

An iron is a great way to make a garment look crisp and presentable. I recommend that you choose an iron with a silver bottom. Irons, which have a black bottom, have been treated with various chemicals which leech into the air when the iron is heated.

Air Purifiers

I also recommend that every home invest in an air purifier, considering the dust, dirt, indoor and outdoor air pollution, which we come in contact with daily.

The best overall air purifier I have come across is The Filter Queen. Sharper Image **www.filterqueen.com** also carries some options for air purifiers **www.sharperimage.com/si**

Kitchen and Bathroom

One of the keys to a healthy lifestyle is to not create issues based on the choices you make. One key is in the areas of reducing or preventing mold, mildew and bacteria.

In your bathroom and kitchen, NEVER leave dishrags, towels, sponges etc. lying in a heap. Always lay folded once or flat over a bar or faucet. Also when using a dishcloth or wash cloth, they can be cleaned regularly with **Nature's Gate** tea tree shampoo or Miracle Mineral Solutions which helps to kill germs! This can also be used as shower gel. Never use toxic synthetics to clean kitchen and bathrooms. **Seventh Generation** carries a line of natural products for kitchen and bathroom.

Proper Ventilation – Leave bathroom door and windows cracked while showering/bathing. Moisture and steam create mold, mildew and bacteria.

Water Treatment Systems

My recommendation as one of the best water treatment systems that I have come across is the Kangen alkaline water system. Kangen alkaline water filters out toxic chemicals such as heavy metals, chlorine, fluoride and other toxins. Once this is done, essential trace minerals are then released in the water.

My health has been improved greatly, since I started drinking this water! I found that I had an improved skin complexion, clearer skin, increased energy, better absorption, hydration, better elimination and so many more benefits!

I have found numerous benefits to drinking this water. You can do a bit of research and hear numerous testimonials of how this has helped to improve the health and well-being of many people around the world!

To research this, I suggest you go to the website: **www.enagic.com**

Upgrading shower heads with filters

In straight tap water, there are numerous toxins readily present. While we more often will eliminate them in our diet, we can often neglect these with the water used for showering or taking a bath. I strongly implore you to purchase a shower head that specifically filters these toxins out. Visit your local health food store and purchase there.

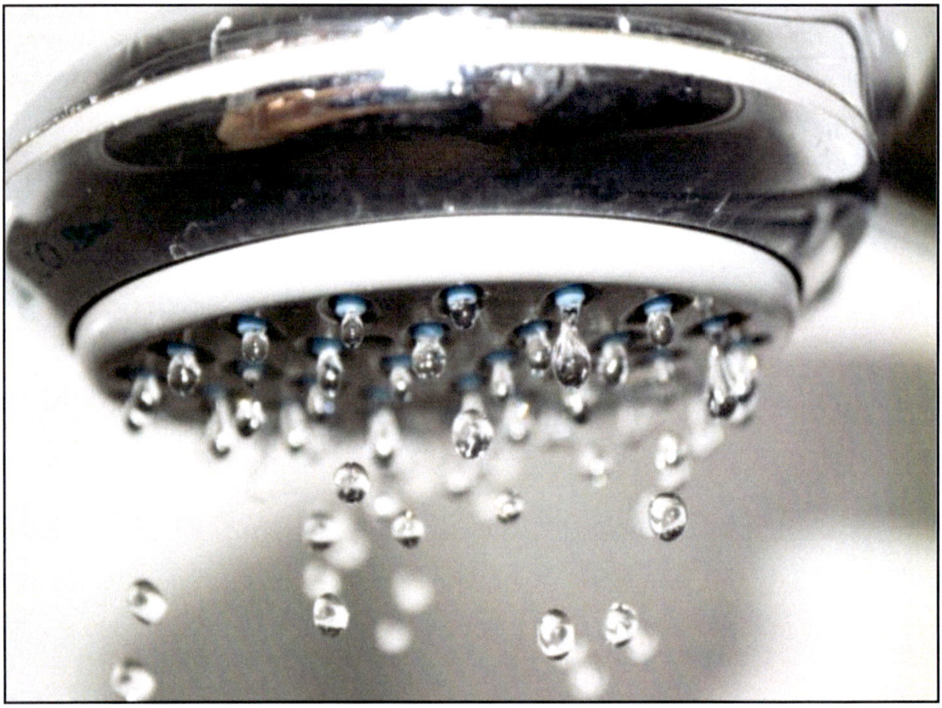

Caring for Our Outdoors

We all must take responsibility for the air we breathe! A true commitment means growing your own garden along with better management of your yard.

I strongly recommend that you do not spray any chemicals on your lawn; so that, we can work in harmony with earth's eco-system. We actually need important bugs, insects and bees for pollinating our flowers and fruit. Common weeds like dandelions along with other root and herbs, are actually edible from organic soil that has not been sprayed.

An option to consider is to maintain your grass using an electric lawn mower with a mulching blade. Many retailers, including **Home Depot, Lowes** and **Sears,** carry a wide variety from which to choose. Electric lawnmowers are highly efficient and come with their own batteries, which can be recharged! They have minimal waste and bi-products. So, using one reduces pollution, saves money and eliminates the need to use gas and oil. I absolutely love them!

Selecting and Caring for Your Vehicle

Buy a hybrid or electric vehicle

Another key area to consider if we want fresh and clean air is to consider the type of vehicle we drive.

Hybrid and electric vehicles are becoming more popular, as many people are becoming more aware of the many benefits of driving them.

Benefits include: Eco-friendly, low emissions, saves on gas, helps to improve the lives of all life forms, including humans, animals, wild life etc. by reducing pollution!

Hybrid Vehicles

Perhaps the most convenient vehicle at this time (environmentally speaking), is to consider purchasing or leasing a hybrid vehicle. This may be the most convenient choice for now. Car brands which carry hybrid vehicles include: **Chevy, Buick, Nissan, KIA, Honda, Hyundai, and BMW.** I practically favor the **Nissan Leaf** and the median price range for this vehicle is $25,000.

Electric Vehicles

Wouldn't it be cool, if we never had to stop for gas again and instead of gas stations, we have car charging stations that are much lower in price! I love this idea! This would be Awesome and we will improve the quality of our air! This may be our reality in the near future, as the consciousness of this concept continue to raise! This type of vehicle requires no gas only charging like charging your cellular phone, only it's a larger unit. Generally most electric cars require charging every 70-80 miles and can be plugged in overnight using a charging station in your garage while you sleep! Electric cars are on the market now and if you are a city driver, perhaps you could purchase an electric car if you drive less than 70 miles in a given day or you could have one as a second vehicle! There is however a top of the line electric vehicle that can be driven up to 280 miles and is a **Tesla** vehicle. There are also other things to consider, when purchasing an electric car, so do your research!

Also keep in mind if you would like a hybrid or electric vehicle; you may need to special order it.

Envirotabs

Increase gas mileage and decrease emissions (pollution) with Envirotabs. Users report that they have seen noticeable results with cars greater than five years old. Cars that are newer can also benefit. For more information visit: **www.greenfootglobal.com**

Other considerations

While riding in a vehicle, when you are not defogging windows, it's a good idea to keep circulating air within the vehicle, instead of taking in from outside. You do not want to breathe in more toxic chemicals. You will also keep any warm or cool air re-circulating in the car which means the temperature of the inside will be more of what you want.

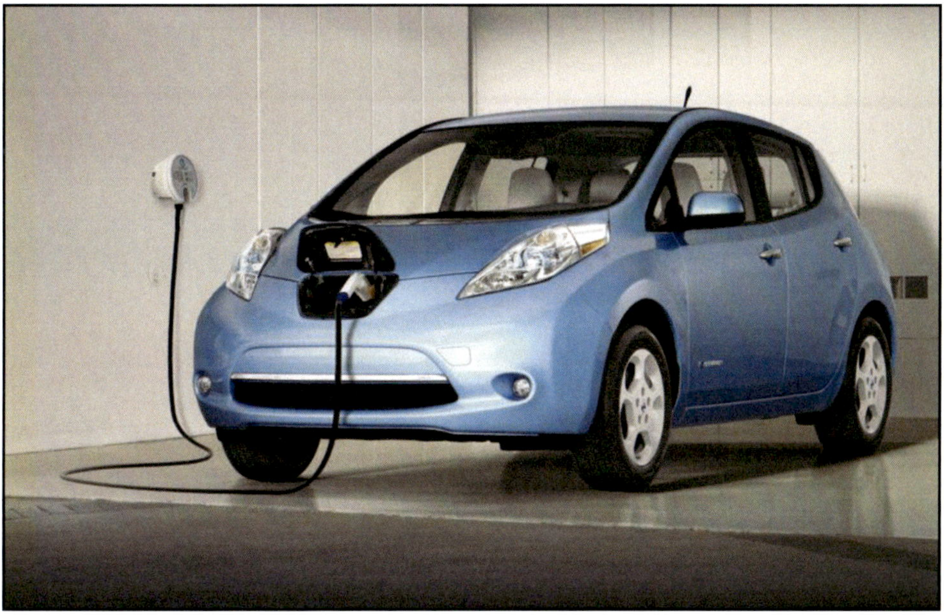

Helpful things to Eliminate/ Reduce from Your Lifestyle

(Be sure to read labels on all of these)

- ❑ Aerosols
- ❑ Artificial Sweeteners and Preservatives
- ❑ Boxed foods (processed)
- ❑ Candles (becomes toxic when lit, including soy)
- ❑ Canned Foods
- ❑ Cell phones- use an earpiece when talking (reduce talk time when without earpiece)
- ❑ Chemical based Household Cleaners
- ❑ Commercial deodorants
- ❑ Commercial dish detergent
- ❑ Commercial laundry detergent
- ❑ Commercial lotions and body oils
- ❑ Frozen dinners
- ❑ Hair dye and rinses (see alternative)
- ❑ Incenses (diffuse essential oils instead)
- ❑ Microwave (use toaster oven)
- ❑ Negative Toxic People
- ❑ Perfume, Fragrances and Nail Polish (very toxic)
- ❑ Plug-ins and air fresheners
- ❑ Quit Smoking
- ❑ Reduce Stress
- ❑ Relaxers/Perms (see alternatives)
- ❑ Soda pop (loaded with sugar, diet isn't any better either)

❑ Teflon cookware and utensils (see alternatives)
❑ Commercial Skincare
❑ Check off and date as you reduce or eliminate these items!

Items To Release

This book is helping you with a Wellness Makeover! What you discard is totally up to you. You may also choose to give things away instead to someone who may find them useful.

Optional: You may want to share with others why you are releasing them from your diet and lifestyle. Have you ever thought about how much plastic you use and if it's necessary? Think about this, instead of buying storage bags, you could use containers that can be used over and over again. This saves you money and part of the solution of reducing waste.

Here are a few suggestions:

❑ Purchase glass containers with lids and re-use your jars from food purchases.
❑ If you must use plastic, make it a habit to not purchase it.
❑ Only use it if you purchased something in it previously and save it to use over again!

Reusable Items

❑ Glass containers
❑ Plastic containers

Recyclable Items

❑ Soda pop cans
❑ Aluminum
❑ Metal
❑ Cellular phones
❑ Microwaves
❑ Glass
❑ Cardboard ❑ Styrofoam ❑ Plastic

Where to Recycle

Clean items may be recycled at the following places:

- ❏ Your curbside

Local recycling facility or stores such as:

❏ Target:	Cell phones
❏ Best Buy:	CD's and DVD's

Your Commitment

This is your commitment to bring order and harmony to your living space and make it in line with your new vision for yourself. Make an outline here of changes that you are going to initiate.

Changes in my home which I give myself permission to make include:

____

____

____

Items I am excited to invest in for myself and my health include:

____

____

____

A change which is a stretch, but I know I can do is:

____

____

____

I am at peace with these decisions I am making because:

____

____

Lotus Life

My Final Thoughts

Thank you for allowing me to introduce these changes in your awareness. I appreciate the opportunity to share with you my story as well as my experiences.

Perhaps in the near future, we will start to see more people become more conscious of what they consume and want to take better care of their health. With this rise in awareness, we will start to see more people planting their own gardens and more chain health food stores all over the country and all over the world.

There is a time where the student becomes the teacher. I encourage you to become a student of the choices you want to make. Keep this as a first point of reference; also read, research, look online, talk to farmers, store owners, diners and people whom you see doing this. Write down your experiences and keep a health journal.

If you find a great recipe, a wonderful product or a success strategy, I want you to let me know. I am always learning and growing in my knowledge and experiences and I can share it with my other students/clients, and gladly give you credit. It is my sincere hope that this book has been a blessing to you and that you will always choose what is best for you; concerning your health and well-being. Another one of the greatest gifts that the Creator has given us is free will. I encourage you to use it to make better choices for yourself, your family, your future and our planet starting today!

Thank you for taking the time and investing in Awaken to Natural Health!
~Namaste

Katina Love

Recommendations

Books:

These can be found either on-line or in your favorite bookstore:

- Gentle Babies, by: Debra Rayburn
- Natural Cures they don't want ou to know about, by Kevin Trudeu
- Living Balanced, by: Stacey Kimbrell
- Recipes for Longer Life, by: Ann Wigmore
- Essential Oils Pocket Reference, 5th Edition
- Fountain of Youth, by: Peter Kelder
- You can Heal your Life, by: Louise L. Hay
- Getting into the Vortex Meditations, Also audio, by: Abraham Hicks

Videos:

Learn about breast feeding: **www.youtube.com/watch?v=Yr0sbmzmV9k/**

Websites:

- Alkaline Water system: **www.enagic.com**
- Learn about essential oils. The Missing Link: **www.youtube.com**
- Learn about testimonials. Type: Essential oils testimonials: **www.youtube.com**
- Your diet and blood type: **www.dadamo.com**
- Music Therapy to help with memory: **musicandmemory.org**
- Probiotic Drink: **www.synergydrinks.com**
- Learn about Apple Cider Vinegar: **www.bragg.com**
  Learn about & order, Miracle Solution (MMS): **www.mmsdrops.com/great-home-uses-for-mms**
- Order Nutri-bullet: **www.nutribullet.com**
- Order wheatgrass & juicing machine: **www.wheatgrasshome.com**
- Shop for quality cotton clothes: **www.aummygoddessstore.com**
- Save money on gas: **greenfootglobal.com**
- Types of air filters: **www.filterqueen.com** and **www.sharperimage.com/si**
- Nutrition data: **www.nutritiondata.self.com**
- Free on-line diet, weight loss journal and up to date tips: **www.fitday.com**